Homeopathy
for Women

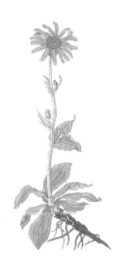

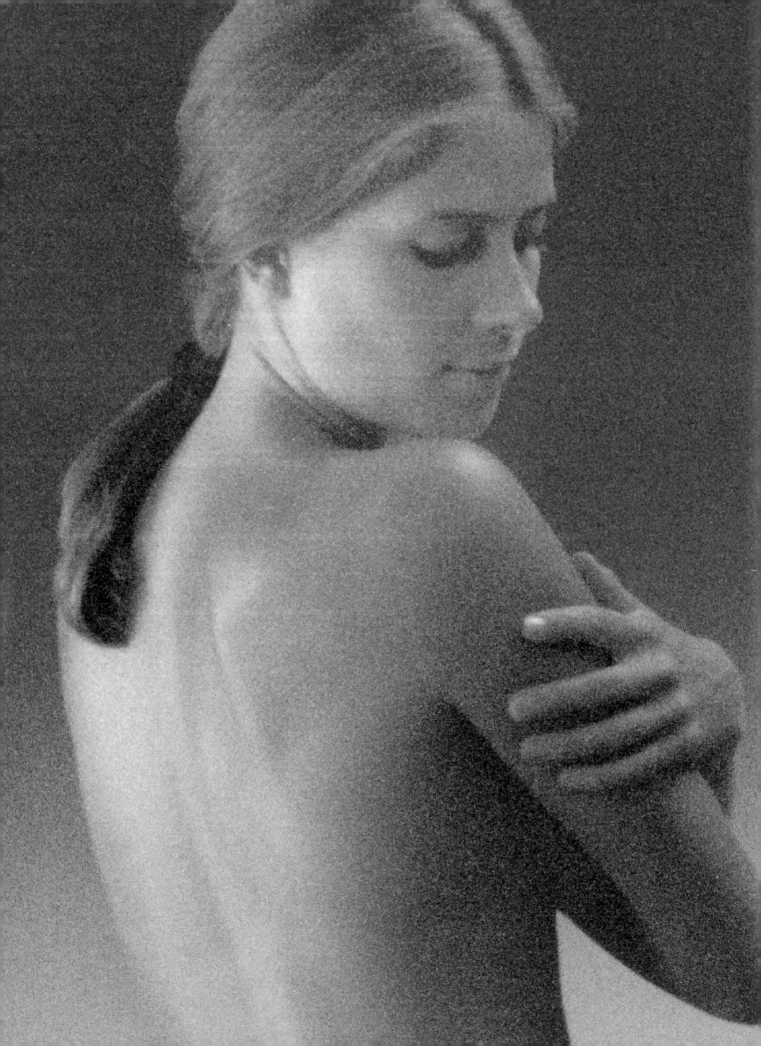

Homeopathy
for Women

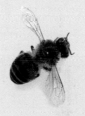

A comprehensive, easy-to-use guide for women of all ages

Dr BARRY ROSE MRCS LRCP DRCOG FFHom *and*
Dr CHRISTINA SCOTT-MONCRIEFF MB ChB MFHom

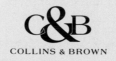

COLLINS & BROWN

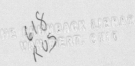

First published in Great Britain in 1998
by Collins & Brown Limited
London House
Great Eastern Wharf
Parkgate Road
London SW11 4NQ

1 3 5 7 9 8 6 4 2

British Library Cataloguing-in-Publication Data:
A catalogue record for this book
is available from the British Library.

ISBN 1 85028 392 3

Editor: Mary Lambert
Design: The Bridgewater Book Company
Photography: Ian Parsons except p69, 86 top, 93, 136 by Zul Makhida
Illustrator: Michael Courtney
American text: Dr Jacquelyn Wilson

Reproduction by HBM Print Pte Ltd, Singapore
Printed and bound in Italy by L.E.G.O.

Contents

P A R T O N E

AILMENTS

CHAPTER I

THE BREASTS, REPRODUCTIVE & URINARY SYSTEMS
page 14

CHAPTER 2

PREGNANCY, BIRTH & POST-PARTUM PROBLEMS
page 32

CHAPTER 3

THE MENOPAUSE
page 50

CHAPTER 9

EMOTIONAL PROBLEMS
page 116

CHAPTER 10

EMERGENCIES
page 134

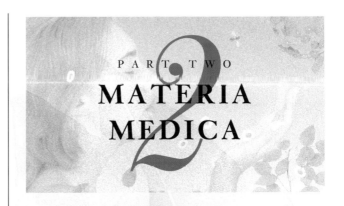

PART TWO

MATERIA MEDICA
2

CHAPTER 11

COMMON HOMEOPATHIC MEDICINES
page 146

Foreword

I first developed an interest in homeopathy when, as a medical student, I began to realize that a lot of illnesses were preventable. Although our mind and our body are our most valuable assets, from time to time we subject them to extreme and often unnecessary abuse. Some of this is unavoidable; planetary pollution is a fast-growing fact of life, worry, stress and anxiety are always present and we often eat substances to which we are allergic or sensitive, and that are therefore bad for us. However, I started to wonder whether the very substances we were using to treat diseases were perhaps adding to these hazards and that the medicines that we were using to 'cure' illnesses were not as safe as we thought. I began to explore avenues other than those of orthodox medicine to see if there was any truth in this.

While I was training as a conventional doctor, I realized that, at times, modern drugs have become implicated in this process of abuse. It is almost as if they are too good. They are so powerful that, paradoxically, they often have multiple side-effects that can disturb systems of the body other than the ones for which they are being given. In other words they too can cause illness. Sometimes the effects of the patient's initial illness far outweigh the risks of the side-effects of the drugs used and in this situation one has to make a conscious decision as to what to do. However, as a homeopathic doctor, I can use another method of treatment that is safe, free of side-effects and for many illnesses, restores health quickly and gently. It is not, however, a panacea and has to be used responsibly, as does any form of treatment.

Homeopathy is a branch of complementary medicine. *It has been called this rather than* alternative *because it is perfectly safe to use, not only on its own instead of orthodox medicine, but also, when necessary, in conjunction with it. There is never any contra-indication to using the two systems, conventional and homepathic, together. When they are used in this way, it is frequently found that a considerably lower dose of the conventional drug may be given. Naturally, whenever possible, I use homeopathic medicines alone and have found over many years in practice that a very high percentage of cases can be managed with purely homeopathic treatment.*

A few of the conditions mentioned in this book are not suitable for complete self-medication but, even in these cases, homeopathic treatment can be started while waiting to see your doctor or can be given in conjunction with your doctor's prescription. Many doctors these days accept that homeopathy has something to offer in the treatment of illness and are not unhappy about you using it.

Finally, like all things, practice makes perfect and the more you use homeopathic medicine, the more confidence you will gain in its use. In this way, proof of its ability to act in treating illness will be there for you to see and feel.

Dr Barry Rose MRCS LRCP DRCOG FFHom

Introduction

HOMEOPATHIC MEDICINES have been used for some 200 years to treat a wide variety of illnesses safely and effectively. The word homeopathy means 'like suffering'. It describes the basic principle of homeopathic treatment: that the symptoms that a person experiences can be cured by a substance that would cause the same symptoms if given to a healthy person. This principle was recognized by Hippocrates 2,400 years ago, but it was not used in a systematic way until Dr Samuel Hahnemann (1755–1843) grew tired of the brutal medical practices of his day and began to experiment with other forms of treatment.

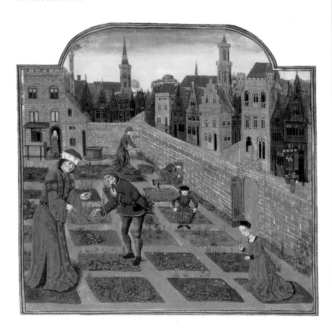

Even back in medieval times the power of herbs to help cure illnesses was realized. Often they were grown in gardens, such as this town garden, to be used for medicinal purposes.

Using herbs, and later other substances including the medicines of the day, such as arsenic and mercury, Hahnemann gathered a group of healthy people who took the substance he was investigating, and then reported their symptoms. These were called 'provings' and were recorded. They became the basis of the prescriptions Hahnemann later gave to ill people with the same symptoms.

Taking medicines that caused the same symptoms that a patient was already experiencing sometimes caused an *aggravation* of the symptoms. To overcome this, Hahnemann devised a method of preparing the medicine by systematically diluting the original medicine, or 'mother tincture', and shaking it vigorously between each dilution. To his surprise, this method enhanced the action of the medicine. He called the method 'potentisation' and the resulting medicines '*potencies*', thus the highest potencies contain the weakest solutions.

Hahnemann's method is still used today. The mother tincture is diluted on one of two scales: either one part in ten, or one part in 100. The number of dilutions that a medicine has undergone is recorded on each bottle of medicine by a number, which is usually printed just after the name of the medicine. The dilution scale is indicated by a letter, so x or d means that each dilution was one part in ten and c denotes dilutions of one part in 100. For example, a medicine which has 6c on it means that the mother tincture has been diluted by one part in a hundred six times. A 1000c dilution is usually denoted as 1M.

Giving such small doses has always been controversial because the original substance must eventually disappear altogether. Modern chemistry tells us that this occurs at about the 12c dilution, so how can the higher potencies be effective? It is thought the medicine leaves some sort of message in the water during the vigorous shaking between dilutions, and that this message somehow resonates with the body to promote healing.

The Vital Force

Hahnemann believed that the body contains an innate power to heal itself. He called this the Vital Force. He believed that when a person is ill this force becomes disordered and that homeopathic medicines are able to restore it in a unique way. The choice of medicine depends on the symptoms that are present and is called the *symptom medicine* in this book. The term local medicine is sometimes also used.

In more long-standing illnesses, the Vital Force may put up a good resistance to the progress of the disease, but over a period of time the illness becomes more severe. Symptom medicines may bring some relief, but they rarely cure this type of illness and a *constitutional medicine* may be needed. Such a prescription is based on the whole personality and appearance of the patient.

How to use this book

Part one of this book contains information about the problems and ailments that women may encounter during their lives. Each chapter has an introduction that provides more useful information and there are self-help tips. Part two is the *Materia Medica* section where there is a detailed description of 50 common medicines.

To select the most appropriate medicine for your current complaint you should:

≈ Use the list of book contents and/or index to find the entry that most closely describes the problem.

≈ Read through the symptoms to find those that best describe your symptoms so that you can select the most appropriate medicine.

≈ Use the *Materia Medica* section, where possible, to confirm your choice. The introduction to the *Materia Medica* will help you use this section.

≈ You should take the medicine at least half an hour after eating and when your mouth is free of other strong flavors, such as peppermint, toothpaste or tobacco. In an emergency, if you cannot wait, rinse your mouth with water if this is possible.

≈ Allow the medicine to dissolve in your mouth.

Taking a course of treatment

≈ If the symptoms improve, reduce the frequency of the doses of medicine and stop it altogether when you are symptom free. If the symptoms do return, you need to start taking the recommended medicine again.

≈ If any of the symptoms get worse you should stop taking the medicine. Even with the very dilute 'potentised' medicines it is possible that you are 'proving' the medicine or experiencing an aggravation

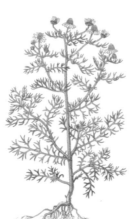

A tincture from the chamomile plant makes the homeopathic medicine Chamomilla.

(see opposite). This is not necessarily a bad sign, because it shows that the medicine is having an effect, and the reaction will almost always subside within a day or two leaving you symptom free. If some of your symptoms persist, try a few doses in a higher potency, but it is a good idea to check whether another medicine might be more appropriate. If in doubt consult a homeopath. If the symptoms are severe, or if you have other health problems, seek medical help.

≈ If some symptoms still remain while others improve, you should take the medicine less frequently, eventually stopping it. You will need to change to a different medicine if some symptoms remain.

≈ If new symptoms appear, stop the medicine. All homeopathic medicines have a wider action than those mentioned in this book and you may be 'proving' the medicine (see opposite). If the symptoms persist consider taking another medicine.

≈ If your symptoms do not change, try to find a more appropriate medicine.

≈ If you are concerned about what is happening always seek professional advice. Remember to consult your doctor *before* you stop any conventional medication or alter the recommended dose. You should also always tell your homeopath what medicines your doctor has prescribed for you.

Further Help

Homeopathic medicines are increasingly available from drugstores and health food stores. Higher potencies and also the less common ones can be bought by mail order from a homeopathic manufacturer using a credit card.

The best way to find a qualified homeopathic doctor is to contact the National Center for Homeopathy which provides a directory of qualified doctors (see page 173). Although a growing number of health care providers prescribe homeopathic medicines, only three states, Nevada, Arizona and Connecticut, have homeopathic licensing boards and require doctors to pass an examination. However, the letters DHt after a doctor's name indicates membership of the specialty board of the American Board of Homeotherapeutics.

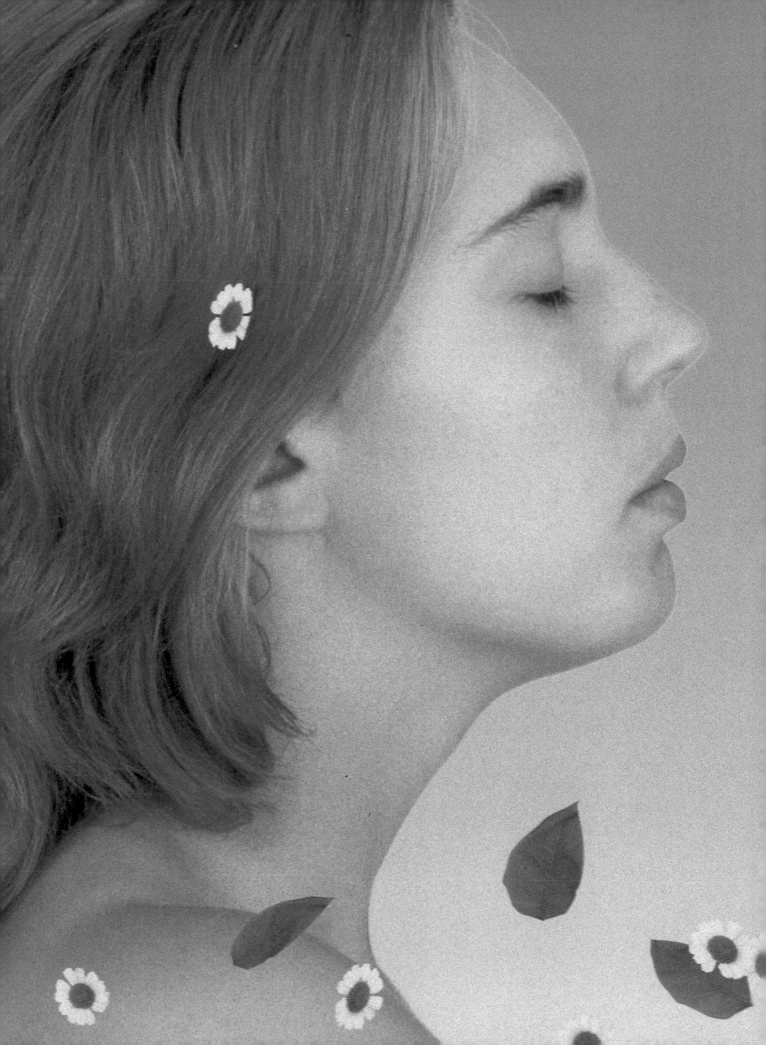

PART ONE

AILMENTS

CHAPTER 1

THE BREASTS, REPRODUCTIVE & URINARY SYSTEMS

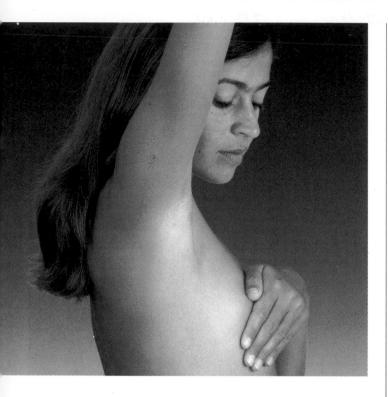

A WOMAN'S BODY undergoes regular changes during the reproductive years because of the monthly variations in hormone levels. Shortly after a period, as the ovaries are preparing to release an egg (ovulation), they secrete the hormone estrogen, which begins to thicken the lining of the uterus (womb) in readiness for a pregnancy, should the egg become fertilized. After ovulation, the ovaries secrete the hormone progesterone, which continues to prepare the uterus to receive the fertilized egg. Hormone levels decrease if the egg is not fertilized, and the egg is shed along with the lining of the uterus during the next monthly period.

Period problems and premenstrual syndrome are common reasons for consulting

Breast pain is a common symptom and is often noticed before a period: the cause is unknown but is thought to be hormonal.

a doctor. These are areas where homeopathy is often useful, but if you are not helped by the medicines that are suggested in this chapter (see also Fibroids, p55), you may need to seek a constitutional prescription.

BREASTS

Female breasts enlarge at puberty under the influence of the sex hormones. Initially one breast may be larger than the other but eventually they are usually much the same size. The size of the breasts, however, changes during the menstrual cycle, during pregnancy and lactation, and after the menopause.

Breast pain is a common symptom and may be at its worst shortly before a period. Unfortunately, the cause is unknown, although it is likely to be some minor irregularity in the control of the sex hormones. If you experience pain, especially if there are nodules or lumps in the breast at the same time, you should consult your doctor, who will usually be able to reassure you. The early stages of breast cancer are very rarely painful.

The main function of the breasts is the production of milk to feed a baby, but they are also regarded as symbols of femininity and beauty. The nipples are very sensitive to touch and contains small muscle fibers that, when they contract, cause the nipple to become erect during sexual arousal or from the cold. Discharge from the nipple that is not related to childbirth or breast-feeding is not a common symptom, and should always be discussed with your doctor.

SEXUAL BEHAVIOUR

Despite the recent acceptance of a much more open approach to sexuality, many women do not find it easy to talk about sexual problems. Some researchers believe

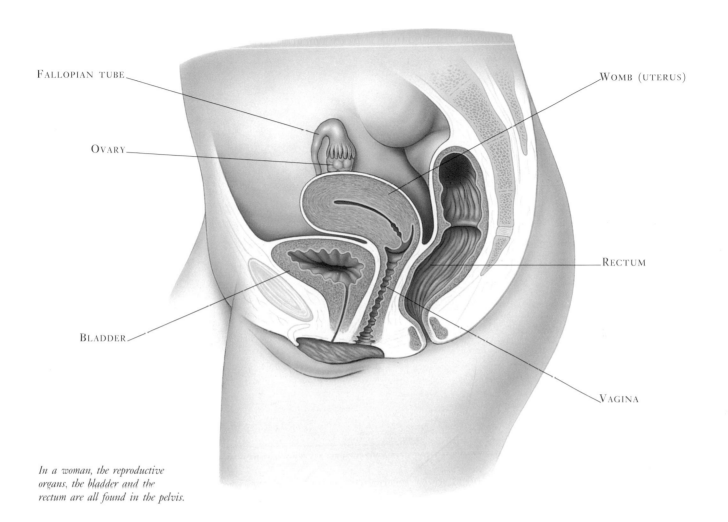

FALLOPIAN TUBE

OVARY

BLADDER

WOMB (UTERUS)

RECTUM

VAGINA

In a woman, the reproductive organs, the bladder and the rectum are all found in the pelvis.

that as many as 50 per cent of marriages are troubled by sexual problems at some stage. Overcoming such problems may be easier if you understand what is generally considered to be normal sexual behavior. This can be divided into four phases:

✥ *Interest or desire* It is normal to have an interest in sex, to seek sexual contact and to experience sexual thoughts and fantasies.

✥ *Arousal or excitement* In this phase there is an increased supply of blood to the genital organs, and the vagina balloons and becomes lubricated. Thoughts and feelings become focused on the sexual experience.

✥ *Orgasm* The walls of the vagina contract rhythmically and there is an intense sensual experience that spreads from the clitoris throughout the body.

✥ *Resolution* The physical changes gradually reverse.

There are many women whose sexual life and experience differs from the so-called normal pattern just described. If you and your partner are content with your sex life you should not worry if it appears to differ from that of other people.

VAGINAL DISCHARGE

During the reproductive years the cervix and the walls of the vagina secrete mucus which is then discharged from the vagina. The amount of discharge and its nature varies not only from woman to woman but also at different phases of the menstrual cycle. Most women notice an increased discharge after sexual arousal, even if sexual intercourse has not taken place, and during pregnancy. The oral contraceptive pill can also change the amount of discharge. Any abnormal change in your discharge should always be discussed with your doctor as 80 per cent of cases are the result of an infection. Other causes include erosions or polyps of the cervix, incomplete miscarriages or retained placenta and forgotten tampons. All these causes require conventional medical treatment, but where no obvious physical cause is found, homeopathic treatment can be very helpful.

SEXUALLY TRANSMITTED DISEASES (STDS)

The epidemic of STDs that started in the 'Swinging Sixties' is now gradually declining thanks to the increased use of condoms as a means of avoiding the risk of AIDS. The Pill did away with the need for barrier methods of birth control, which had given protection against STDs. It also gave women easy control of their own fertility and as a result they have become more likely to have a greater number of sexual partners. However, for many women STDs have led to blocked or damaged fallopian tubes, which can cause problems with conception and also an increased likelihood of ectopic (tubal) pregnancies (see page 42).

Genital warts and herpes are often sexually transmitted. The warts need to be treated because there is concern that some strains of the virus may cause cervical cancer. Conventional treatment is the careful application of special (not over-the-counter) wart preparations, but this cannot be done during pregnancy. The homeopathic treatment is constitutional, but there are a few specific remedies that may be worth trying if you are pregnant or while you are waiting for other treatment.

Genital herpes is caused by one of the *Herpes simplex* viruses (HSV). The two strains of this virus – HSV-1 and HSV-2 – can both cause genital herpes, but HSV-1 is more frequently found in cold sores on the lips and face, from where it can cause genital sores after oral-genital contact. The first attack of genital herpes is usually the most severe, and your doctor is likely to prescribe antiviral therapy. Recurrent episodes are usually less severe but you should remember that

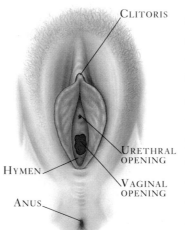

CLITORIS

URETHRAL OPENING

HYMEN

VAGINAL OPENING

ANUS

Inflammation of the bladder or urethra can cause pain when passing urine.

you can pass on the infection whenever lesions are present. Herpes can also be fatal to babies, and a Caesarean section is likely to be recommended if lesions are active in late pregnancy. Both homeopathic constitutional and symptom treatments can help.

CYSTITIS

The word 'cystitis' means inflammation of the bladder. The earliest known prescriptions for its treatment were inscribed on an Egyptian papyrus over 3,000 years ago.

The most common symptom is pain when passing urine. This can be relatively mild or excruciating. Because the bladder is irritated, the sensation of 'wanting to go' often occurs before the bladder is as full as usual, and most women feel that the bladder is not completely emptied even when they have just been to the toilet. Some women with cystitis also pass blood with their urine. Cystitis is commonly caused by infection and this can usually be cured with a short course of antibiotics. However, homeopathy can be extremely useful to treat the symptoms while a woman waits for the result of a urine culture. Cystitis rarely causes fever, but if this does occur, especially if there is also pain in the kidney region, medical advice is essential.

THE URETHRAL SYNDROME

Easy access to laboratory diagnosis of urinary infection has alerted doctors to the fact that as many as half of women with cystitis symptoms do not have a bacterial infection, but are experiencing irritation in the urethra. The urethra is the short tube that connects the bladder to the outside and lies very close to the vagina. Urethral irritation can follow sexual intercourse, when there has been some minor bruising, or can be caused by vaginal infection. Homeopathic medicines can be extremely useful.

If you suffer from regular bouts of cystitis symptoms, you may be helped by the suggestions discussed on page 17.

CYSTITIS

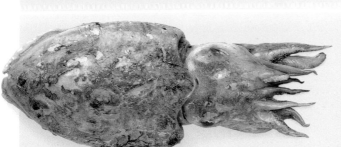

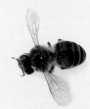

PULSATILLA

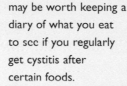

CUTTLEFISH
(SEPIA IS PREPARED FROM THE
INK OF THE CUTTLEFISH)

HONEY BEE
(*APIS MELLIFICA* IS DERIVED
FROM THE HONEY BEE.)

Various homeopathic remedies can be used to help the unpleasant symptoms of cystitis.

RELIEVING THE SYMPTOMS OF CYSTITIS

- Start taking your homeopathic medicine (see page 18).
- Drink 570ml/1 pint of water, and then aim to drink a further 290ml/½ pint every half hour. This helps to wash out the germs.
- Relieve the symptoms by making your urine alkaline. To do this, add 5ml/1 teaspoonful of sodium bicarbonate to your drinking water every 6 hours. (Avoid vitamin C and cranberry juice: these make the urine acid.)
- Get into a warm bath or fill a hot water bottle with warm water and put it on your lower abdomen or between the thighs.

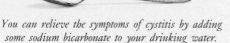

You can relieve the symptoms of cystitis by adding some sodium bicarbonate to your drinking water.

WHEN TO CONSULT A DOCTOR

- If the symptoms do not improve in 24 hours with these self-help measures.
- If you are feverish.
- If the pain moves to the kidneys.

AVOIDING RECURRENT ATTACKS OF CYSTITIS

- Always drink lots of water: 1.5–2.5 litres/3–5 pints a day.
- Wear cotton panties.
- Let the air circulate around the perineal area by avoiding tight trousers and wearing open-crotch tights. If possible, use tampons rather than sanitary pads.

- Shower instead of bathing. If you do have a bath, do not stay in for a long soak or add bath salts or antiseptics to the water.
- Never use soap on the perineum.
- Avoid vaginal douches or deodorants.
- After movement of the bowels wipe yourself from front to back to avoid infection, or use a bidet.
- Always empty your bladder before and after sexual intercourse to flush out the germs that cause cystitis, and can double in number every 20 to 30 minutes.
- Drink cranberry juice as a preventive measure (but see advice, left). The germs like to attach themselves to the bladder wall and cranberry juice seems to act by making the lining of the bladder too slippery.
- In a few women, the symptoms of cystitis are caused by food intolerance. If you are prone to cystitis and suffer from other allergies, it may be worth keeping a diary of what you eat to see if you regularly get cystitis after certain foods.

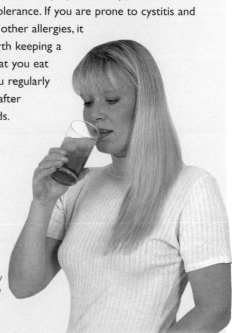

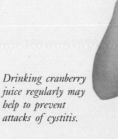

Drinking cranberry juice regularly may help to prevent attacks of cystitis.

Acute cystitis

Almost all women will have sudden attacks of acute cystitis and/or the urethral syndrome from time to time (see page 16). While recurrent attacks of cystitis should always be investigated, you may be helped by one of the following medicines.

SYMPTOMS / MEDICINE

Symptoms	Medicine
❧ Frequent urination with burning, stinging pain in the bladder. ❧ Urine passed in small amounts. ❧ Lack of thirst. ❧ A tendency to swollen hands and feet.	◉ Apis mellifica
❧ Sudden onset of symptoms. ❧ Severe, incapacitating burning pain, that is worst while urine is being passed. ❧ The urine is often bloodstained.	◉ Cantharis
❧ Onset is less intense, but there may be blood in the urine at an early stage. ❧ Symptoms are worse at night. ❧ May be indicated if excessive saliva is produced.	◉ Mercurius corrosivus
❧ Bad pain and an urge to urinate. ❧ A feeling that it 'cannot be stood': want help *now*. ❧ Pain worse before and shortly after urination. ❧ Much better for warmth, especially a warm bath.	◉ Nux vomica
❧ Pain is worst at end of urination. ❧ Burning urination and a frequent urge to urinate occurs.	◉ Sarsaparilla
❧ Symptoms start after sexual intercourse or after a catheter has been passed into the bladder. ❧ A feeling that a drop of urine remains in the urethra even after urination.	◉ Staphysagria

DOSAGE

USE THE 30C POTENCY. TAKE EVERY HALF HOUR FOR UP TO TEN DOSES. STOP WHEN THE SYMPTOMS IMPROVE, BUT REPEAT LATER IF NECESSARY.

Chronic cystitis

Many women suffer from milder recurrent (chronic) bladder problems, including an urge to urinate, discomfort during urination, bladder pain and incontinence. Incontinence is an embarrassing topic and few women wish to discuss it, even with their doctors, but almost half of all women over the age of 25 are occasionally incontinent, and one in ten women has a serious problem.

If you are regularly incontinent, consult your doctor as the problem can often be cured, or at least improved. Help can also be obtained from various associations. If you have symptoms of chronic cystitis, you should check with your doctor, in case you need a course of antibiotics, before trying the homeopathic medicines suggested here or for stress incontinence (see page 59).

DOSAGE

USE THE 12C POTENCY. TAKE TWICE A DAY FOR UP TO TWO WEEKS, THEN STOP. REPEAT AS AND WHEN NECESSARY.

SYMPTOMS / MEDICINE

Symptoms	Medicine
❧ Painful urging. ❧ Burning pain after urination and the bladder does not feel empty. ❧ Urge to pass urine in the night.	◉ Lycopodium clavatum
❧ Bladder pain that is worse after urinating or if urination is delayed. ❧ Copious urine occurs, even when not thirsty. ❧ Involuntary urination happens, especially in pregnancy, worse when coughing.	◉ Pulsatilla
❧ A leak of urine occurs when laughing, sneezing or coughing. ❧ There is frequent urinating and sudden urging. ❧ Pain in the lower abdomen if urination is delayed.	◉ Sepia

Breast lumps and mastitis

A tender lumpiness may arise in one or both breasts during early pregnancy, or occasionally at the time of a period. This is normally hormone-induced and is not serious. If the breast becomes tender and redness develops over the painful area, either a breast abscess is about to form or, if you are lactating, acute mastitis is present. Simple, non-malignant lumps do frequently develop in the breast, as do simple cysts, but *medical diagnosis is essential when any lump or cyst is discovered in the breast.*

SYMPTOMS / MEDICINE

Symptoms	Medicine
❧ Mastitis occurs after a chill.	❧ Aconitum napellus
❧ Red streaks radiate from a central point in the breast. ❧ Pulsating pain with hardness of the breast. ❧ A sudden headache often accompanies the mastitis.	❧ Belladonna
❧ Pain occurs because of bruising.	❧ Bellis perennis
❧ The breast is hard to the touch, heavy and painful. ❧ Mastitis occurs after a chill. ❧ Stitching pains and tense swelling are experienced.	❧ Bryonia
❧ Tender and swollen breasts occur before a period.	❧ Calcarea carbonica
❧ Piercing pain which is worse at night. ❧ Tenderness of the rest of the breast, which feels hard. ❧ The breast is painful, even from the touch of clothes or when out walking.	❧ Conium maculatum
❧ Painful, cracked nipples.	❧ Graphites
❧ Chronic mastitis (*medical diagnosis essential*).	❧ Silicea

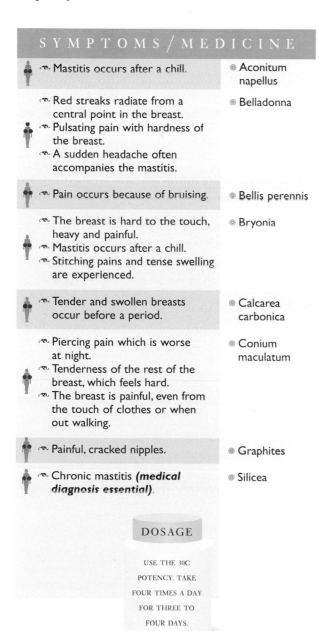

DOSAGE

USE THE 30C POTENCY. TAKE FOUR TIMES A DAY FOR THREE TO FOUR DAYS.

Decreased sexual desire

There are many reasons – psychological, physical – why some women cannot experience sexual pleasure. Loss of sex drive can occur with certain drugs, particularly tranquilizers and anti-hypertensives, and with some diseases, such as diabetes, pelvic disorders, hypothyroidism, multiple sclerosis and muscular dystrophy. Painful intercourse may be an factor. Psychological causes can be inadequate sexual stimulation, anger, fear, guilt, marital discord and stress. Poor arousal technique by the male can lead to the woman's inability to experience sexual satisfaction and can female frigidity. (See page 15.) *Seek medical advice if there is no early response to homeopathic treatment.*

DOSAGE

USE THE 12C POTENCY. TAKE THREE TIMES A DAY UNTIL AN IMPROVEMENT OCCURS. TAKE THEREAFTER IF THE SYMPTOMS RECUR.

SYMPTOMS / MEDICINE

Symptoms	Medicine
❧ An abhorrence of intercourse. ❧ Mental depression occurs.	❧ Agnus castus
❧ Painful intercourse with vaginal burning and soreness. ❧ Feelings of both listlessness and apathy.	❧ Berberis vulgaris
❧ An aversion to intercourse. ❧ A pale, thin, profuse vaginal discharge occurs.	❧ Graphites
❧ Total frigidity. ❧ Great mood changes. ❧ Feels both sensitive and easily excitable.	❧ Ignatia amara
❧ Dry, painful vagina makes intercourse painful.	❧ Lycopodium clavatum
❧ No sexual desire. ❧ Breasts ache and nipples itch. ❧ Tendency to suffer from migraine.	❧ Onosmodium virginianum
❧ Painful vagina on intercourse. ❧ A bearing-down sensation in the pelvis. ❧ Periods are late, scanty and irregular. ❧ Sadness, irritability and indifference felt towards the family.	❧ Sepia

Increased sexual desire

*T*he need to satisfy sexual feelings has no normal standards. So when one woman desires sexual intercourse daily, another might be satisfied with one to two times a week or less. Therefore what is excessive for one individual may be completely normal for another. Feelings of guilt may develop if this increased need for sex leads to promiscuous activity by the individual involved (see also page 15).

SYMPTOMS / MEDICINE

Symptoms	Medicine
• Genital itching with soreness and swelling. • Bloodstained discharge occurs between periods. • Suited to nervous, hypersensitive women.	◉ Ambra grisea
• Burning and itching of the genitalia before and after menstruation. • Increased desire with easy conception.	◉ Calcarea carbonica
• Aching pain over the pelvic area. • Violent backache during the period. • Tendency to be irritable and forgetful.	◉ Calcarea phosphorica
• Fiery sexual desire. • Anxious restlessness. • Early, profuse periods.	◉ Cantharis
• Heavy, frequent, lengthy periods. • Acrid, burning vaginal discharge. • Indifference and avoidance responsibility.	◉ Hydrofluoricum acidum
• Distrustful of others but easily aroused sexually. • A tendency to talk and laugh too much.	◉ Hyoscyamus niger
• Violent sexual excitement is easily brought on by the slightest touch. • Suited to nervous, lively and affectionate women.	◉ Murex purpurea
• Both the external and internal genitalia tingle. • Prone to arrogance and feels contempt for others. • Vaginal spasm occurs.	◉ Platinum metallicum
• A bloodstained discharge is noticed between periods. • Increased sexual drive. • A tendency to miscarriage.	◉ Sabina
• The vulva feels dry, hot and itchy. • Profuse periods accompanied by erotic sensations. • Suited to moody, busy women who are sensitive to music and have a strong sexual desire.	◉ Tarentula hispana

DOSAGE

USE THE 30C POTENCY. TAKE THREE TIMES A DAY FOR ONE WEEK. IT MAY NEED TO BE REPEATED AT MONTHLY INTERVALS UNTIL AN IMPROVEMENT IS MAINTAINED.

Infertility

Failure to conceive

The inability to achieve a pregnancy may be caused by either partner and both should be investigated. The causes of female infertility are numerous and range from congenital defects through the effects of illnesses to psychological problems. Common physical causes are blockage of the fallopian tubes, which prevents the egg produced by the ovary from reaching the uterus (womb), failure of the ovary to produce eggs, vaginal and uterine inflammations, and in some cases vaginal secretion which destroys or damages the male sperm. Anxiety and stress can be factors in the apparent inability to conceive (or, indeed, caused by it), so psychological help and counseling are important. The homeopathic medicines listed below are satisfactory to begin treatment with, but deeper constitutional prescribing is usually necessary.

SYMPTOMS / MEDICINE

Symptoms	Medicine
❧ Great vaginal sensitivity, which may cause spasm and pain before intercourse. ❧ Frequent mental depression which may be severe. ❧ Headaches experienced nightly.	◉ Aurum metallicum
❧ White vaginal discharge that feels warm. ❧ The menstrual period is often early, very profuse and painful, with griping stomach pain extending to the back, plus nausea.	◉ Borax
❧ Heavy periods come too early and last too long. ❧ A milky white vaginal discharge. ❧ Increased sexual desire.	◉ Calcarea carbonica
❧ Intense vaginal irritation. ❧ Periods are offensive, dark and profuse. ❧ A thin, acrid vaginal discharge.	◉ Medorrhinum
❧ Menstrual period is usually late and accompanied by a bearing-down sensation. ❧ Vaginal discharge is irritating and offensive.	◉ Natrum carbonicum
❧ A dry vagina. ❧ Menstrual period is usually irregular and heavy. ❧ A thin, watery, burning vaginal discharge. ❧ Bearing-down pain that is worse in the morning.	◉ Natrum muriaticum
❧ When there has been previous ovarian or fallopian tube inflammation. ❧ Constant tingling and irritation both internally and externally. ❧ Vaginal spasm may make intercourse painful.	◉ Platinum metallicum
❧ A sensation as if all the pelvic organs are dropping. ❧ Green-yellow vaginal discharge. ❧ Periods are late and scanty, or early and heavy. ❧ Intercourse causes vaginal pain.	◉ Sepia

DOSAGE

USE THE 12C POTENCY. TAKE TWICE DAILY FOR ONE MONTH.

Painful intercourse

A number of women who suffer from this condition have no apparent physical abnormalities and it is assumed in these cases (often wrongly) that emotional factors are responsible. A fear of pregnancy is frequently the main cause, although other anxieties and general ill health may be responsible. Some physical causes of this include an intact or tender hymen, a small vaginal canal, vulval inflammation or fissures, vaginal discharges, dryness of the vagina (usually menopausal), tender ovaries, uterine or pelvic tumors, and pelvic inflammatory disease. Painful intercourse often occurs after childbirth, especially if the perineum has become torn. ***All cases need medical advice and diagnosis.***

DOSAGE

USE THE 30C POTENCY. TAKE FOUR TIMES A DAY FOR ONE WEEK.

SYMPTOMS / MEDICINE

Symptoms	Medicine
❧ A swelling of the labia relieved by cold water. ❧ The vagina feels tight. ❧ Soreness and tenderness all over the lower abdomen and pelvic area.	⊛ Apis mellifica
❧ The vagina feels hot and dry. ❧ A sensation as if the contents of the abdomen are about to drop out. ❧ Lower back pain occurs.	⊛ Belladonna
❧ Painful intercourse with vaginal burning and soreness. ❧ Feelings of listlessness and apathy.	⊛ Berberis aquifolium
❧ Bleeding occurs after intercourse. ❧ Burning and soreness of the vagina. ❧ The pelvic organs feel sore and the vulva is itchy, burning and swollen.	⊛ Kreosotum
❧ Dry, painful vagina makes intercourse painful.	⊛ Lycopodium clavatum
❧ The genitalia are hypersensitive with an internal and external tingling sensation. ❧ Vaginal pain and spasm occurs. ❧ Great sexual desire.	⊛ Platina metallicum
❧ The vagina is painful during intercourse. ❧ Prolapse is present, or feels as if it is.	⊛ Sepia

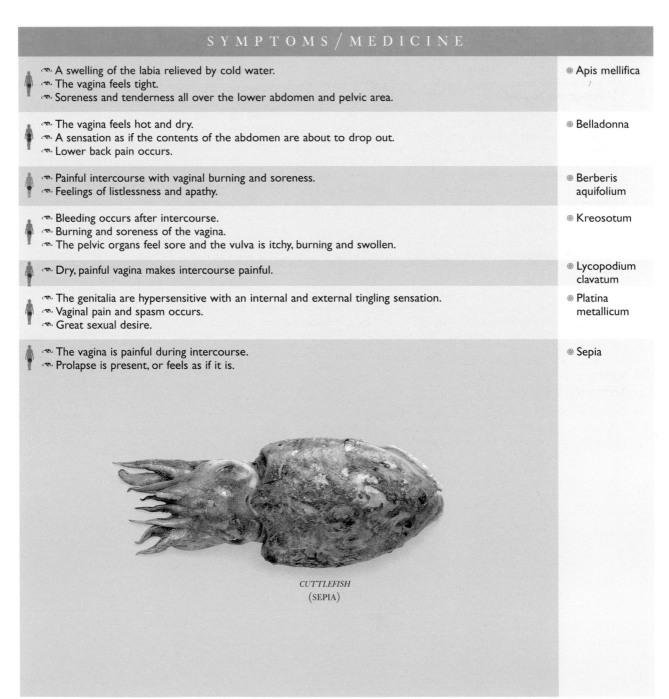

CUTTLEFISH
(SEPIA)

Delayed or absent periods

*T*here may be several causes of these conditions. Primary amenorrhea (the non-appearance of the period at puberty) is usually due to a hormone or endocrine chemical imbalance or to being underweight. Secondary amenorrhea (the disappearance of periods) is commonly due to pregnancy, anorexia nervosa, stress, anemia, endometriosis, polycystic ovaries, starting oral contraception or thyroid hormone deficiency. If you are a very fit athlete, your periods may not start, or they may cease. Either way, you should ensure that your diet is adequate and that you are getting enough calcium. There are other, less common, causes of delayed periods, so if in doubt about what is the cause, seek your doctor's advice.

SYMPTOMS/MEDICINE

Symptoms	Medicine
❧ Feels the cold and suffers from throbbing, suddenly occurring headaches. ❧ Sensation of fullness in the pelvis with a bearing-down sensation. ❧ Urination may be painful.	⊛ Belladonna
❧ The first period is late to commence. ❧ Subsequent periods may occur erratically. ❧ Affects those with a fair complexion and a tendency to perspire easily about the head.	⊛ Calcarea carbonica
❧ Often run-down and tired out. ❧ Prone to palpitations and the ankles can become swollen and puffy. ❧ Flushed complexion and pale and livid with blue margins about the eyes.	⊛ Ferrum metallicum
❧ The first period arrives late. ❧ Once the period commences, it flows on and off, and subsequent periods are very irregular. ❧ The cycle is irregular and often lengthened, especially after getting wet or during emotional stress. ❧ Blood flow may be intermittent.	⊛ Pulsatilla
❧ After a delayed start to the period there is very little loss of blood. ❧ Can be prone to tiredness and have a dark complexion and delicate skin. ❧ A tendency to depression and moodiness, generally better after exertion. ❧ Instead of the period a vaginal discharge may occur at the time that it is due.	⊛ Sepia
❧ A tendency to long cycles. ❧ The first period may be late. ❧ Blood loss is pale and scanty.	⊛ Graphites

DOSAGE

USE THE 30C POTENCY. IF THERE HAS BEEN NO PREVIOUS PERIOD, TAKE THREE TIMES A DAY FOR ONE WEEK AND REPEAT AT MONTHLY INTERVALS UNTIL THE PERIODS BECOME WELL ESTABLISHED. IF THE PERIOD IS DELAYED, TAKE THREE TIMES A DAY, STARTING ON THE DAY THE PERIOD IS DUE.

Heavy periods
Menorrhagia

The average blood loss in a period is 30ml/2 table-spoons, and it is a medical problem until it reaches 80ml/5–6 tablespoons. So the best definition of a heavy period is when it interferes with daily life. There are several causes of heavy menstrual bleeding including fibroids (non-cancerous growths in the uterus), polyps, endometriosis, peri-menopause or a hormonal imbalance. Excessive blood loss each month may lead to anemia. *Heavy vaginal bleeding can signify more serious conditions, so if it occurs monthly, consult a doctor.*

SYMPTOMS/MEDICINE

Symptoms	Medicine
• Early, profuse periods with pain similar to that experienced in early labour. • Extreme fatigue accompanies period. • Period accompanied by indigestion and constipation.	Aletris farinosa
• Bearing-down sensations, which are worse lying down. • Profuse, early, bright red periods. • Cramp-like back pain and cutting pelvic pain.	Belladonna
• Profuse, irregular, long-lasting periods. • Feet feel cold and damp.	Calcarea carbonica
• Bearing-down pain that goes into the thighs. • Flooding occurs.	Calcarea fluorica
• Black, early, profuse periods occur. • Bladder irritation.	Cantharis
• Heavy periods occurring too frequently. • Spasmodic pain accompanies period.	Caulophyllum thalictroides
• Early, profuse periods with backache that moves and muscle ache. • Gloom and dejection accompany period.	Cimicifuga racemosa
• Early, profuse, long-lasting periods. • Body itches during period. • Backache accompanies period.	Kali carbonicum
• Abdominal bloating occurs before period. • Headache and tinnitus accompany period. • Dragging back pain that is relieved by motion. • An acrid, irritating discharge between periods.	Kreosotum
• Dark, thick blood loss that happens chiefly at night.	Magnesia carbonica
• Early, heavy period accompanied by morning nausea and chilliness.	Nux vomica
• Profuse, early, clotted flow. • Great irritation of the genitalia. • Uterine bearing-down sensation. • Heavy periods that occur especially in haughty, melancholic women.	Platinum metallicum

DOSAGE

USE THE 30C POTENCY. TAKE FOUR TIMES A DAY FOR FOUR DAYS, STARTING TWO DAYS BEFORE THE PERIOD IS DUE. IF THE PERIOD IS EARLY, TAKE THE MEDICINE WHEN IT STARTS.

CIMICIFUGA

Irregular periods

The periods are often irregular at the start of puberty, when approaching the menopause and after lactation; this is not abnormal; it is merely an indication of the hormonal changes associated with the particular time of life or condition. In some women, however, the periods never become totally regular. (See also Delayed or absent periods, page 23.)

SYMPTOMS / MEDICINE

- Painful irregular periods with a heavy vaginal discharge between periods.

⊛ Calcarea silicata

- Late to start, the period stops during the night but restarts again the next day.
- A delay in the arrival of the period associated with emotional upsets in a very sympathetic type of woman.

⊛ Causticum

- Pain immediately before the period starts.
- Profuse, dark period with pain that is felt across the pelvis and in the back.
- Skin complaints become worse at the time of the period.

⊛ Cimicifuga racemosa

- The periods, once established, become irregular and delayed.
- Obstinate constipation is a frequent problem.
- Complexion is sallow and frequent, severe headaches may occur.

⊛ Graphites

- Delay in the start of the periods associated with frequent chest infections.

⊛ Kali carbonicum

- Irregular, profuse, frequent periods with large clots occur.
- Breast pain in the duration of a period.
- Violent feelings of sexual excitement.

⊛ Murex purpurea

- Irregular, profuse periods.
- Vagina is dry and there is an acrid, watery vaginal discharge.
- A severe headache develops after the period has finished.

⊛ Natrum muriaticum

- Period is variable both in quantity and timing.
- Fainting and tiredness often accompany period.

⊛ Nux moschata

- Period is always irregular with lower back pain and a desire to defecate.
- Loss of blood is very dark, almost black.

⊛ Nux vomica

- Irregular periods, with a slight, watery blood loss until the next period.
- A feeling of chilliness, but also an intolerance of heat.
- Copious loss of blood which is dark in color.

⊛ Secale cornutum

- A delay in the start of the periods accompanied by an intense backache.
- A delay in the period and it frequently follows a throat or chest infection.

⊛ Senecio aureus

- Period is very slow to start.
- A delay in the onset of the first period in girls who have a clear vaginal discharge which comes on regularly and instead of a normal period.
- Can help those who feel very tired.

⊛ Sepia

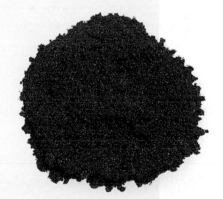

GRAPHITES

DOSAGE

USE THE 30C
POTENCY. TAKE
FOUR TIMES A DAY
FOR THREE DAYS
BEFORE THE PERIOD
IS DUE.

Painful periods
Dysmenorrhea

The pain is largely felt in the back and lower abdomen, and can often be made worse by mental anxiety. Usually coming on a year or two after the start of puberty, there is no known cause, although it is thought that it may be due to a tight cervix (neck of the womb). The pain usually starts just before, or at the start of the period and lasts for about eight to ten hours before it starts to diminish. *If the pain is severe and/or recurrent, see your doctor.*

SYMPTOMS / MEDICINE

Symptoms	Medicine
• Pain comes on before period begins. • A sensation of bearing down, which is worse when lying down but relieved by standing. • Period is profuse and comes early. • Bright red, hot blood loss. • There may be an accompanying cutting pain which goes through the pelvis horizontally. • Period starts and ends quickly. • Unable to bear any kind of jarring.	⊛ Belladonna
• Spasmodic, intermittent bearing-down pains in the groin, and sometimes even in the chest and limbs. • Normal or scanty flow of blood.	⊛ Caulophyllum thalictroides
• Dark, clotted and profuse blood flow. • Pain is intense and spasmodic. • Excessive irritability and impatience.	⊛ Chamomilla
• Pain shoots across the pelvis from side to side and down to the thighs. • Pain starts just before period commences. • During the period, sharp abdominal pains causing doubling up. • Headache develops before beginning of the period.	⊛ Cimicifuga racemosa
• Flow is dark and profuse. • Spasmodic, colicky pains. • Feels weak and tired. • A lot of gas. • Pain is worse at night and may wake the woman up. • Irritability is characteristic. • Severe headache and nausea accompany the period.	⊛ Cocculus indicus
• Severe, left-sided lower abdominal pain and pain from navel to the genital region. • Pain helped by bending double.	⊛ Colocynthis
• Cramp-like pains start before period commences and will continue throughout. • Great relief obtained from warmth, by bending double and from pressure. • Pain is worsened by motion.	⊛ Magnesia phosphorica
• Period is delayed. • Blood flow is dark in color and intermittent. • The more pain, the chillier the woman feels. • Pain seems to move about, causing doubling up, and then causing restlessness and tears.	⊛ Pulsatilla
• Profuse bright loss of blood. • Pain extends into the thighs. • May feel extremely cold with a cold sweat. • Faints from exertion. • Sexual interest is greatly increased just before period.	⊛ Sabina
• Sudden uterine colicky pain develops before period. • Period is often late and the loss is very scanty. • Period may last for only a few hours. • An ache starts in the lower back region and goes down the thighs.	⊛ Veratrum album
• Occasional shooting pains felt in the ovaries. • A violent bearing-down sensation ends in intense cramp, which is felt in the uterus.	⊛ Viburnum opulus
• Pain is agonizing and burning. • Pain extends down thighs, which makes the legs feel as if almost paralyzed. • Blood flow is profuse. • Headache develops over left eye on the day before period.	⊛ Xanthoxylum fraxineum

DOSAGE

USE THE 30C POTENCY. TAKE THREE TIMES A DAY FOR FOUR DAYS BEFORE THE PERIOD IS DUE. IT MAY ALSO BE TAKEN DURING THE PERIOD IF NECESSARY

Premenstrual syndrome *PMS*

*T*his condition, also known as premenstrual tension (PMT), can manifest itself in various ways. For several days before a period starts many women find that they suffer from emotional upsets, such as depression, irritability, loss of sexual desire, extreme anxiety, uncontrollable crying and loss of affection for their family. One or more of these symptoms may be accompanied by weight gain, sore and swollen breasts, swollen ankles and hands, and headache. Additionally there may be some pelvic discomfort and low back pain. As some of these symptoms are related to salt and water retention by the body at this time, simply cutting down (but not cutting out) salt intake will often help.

SYMPTOMS / MEDICINE

❧ Headache which is at its worst on waking. ❧ Face appears, and feels, bloated. ❧ Tight clothes cannot be tolerated, especially around the neck and waist. ❧ Palpitations occur accompanied by a feeling of faintness. ❧ May feel jealous, vindictive, unreasonable and talks excessively, but this improves as soon as the period starts.	◉ Lachesis mutus
❧ As well as feeling irritable, weary, selfish, withdrawn and moody, may have a blinding headache, pallor, nausea and vomiting. ❧ A craving for salt develops before the period. ❧ Abdomen becomes distended, heart feels 'fluttery' and palpitations occur. ❧ The symptoms get worse from noise, mental exertion and consolation, particularly around 10–11 am.	◉ Natrum muriaticum
❧ A lack of thirst is accompanied by a partial loss of sense of taste. ❧ Shooting pain occurs in the neck and upper part of the back. ❧ Very moody and changeable, may cry a lot and want a lot of sympathy. ❧ Symptoms are much improved out of doors.	◉ Pulsatilla
❧ A severe headache. ❧ Food tastes too salty. ❧ A sensation as if the contents of the pelvis are about to drop out. ❧ May feel cold, totally weary and tired, dislike the family, irritable and feel very sad but can liven up with exercise and movement.	◉ Sepia

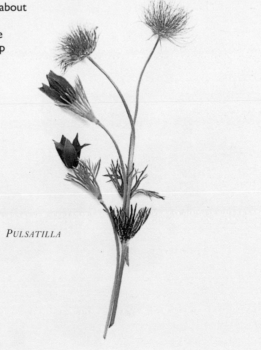

PULSATILLA

Scanty periods

The most common cause of this relatively unimportant condition is the birth control pill. However, it can also occur at one of the three female milestones: adolescence, following pregnancy and around the menopause. Again, at these times it is of little importance, but it can be sometimes be an indication of other illness. *If you feel anything but well, consult a doctor.*

DOSAGE

USE THE 30C POTENCY. TAKE THREE TIMES A DAY FOR THREE DAYS.

SYMPTOMS / MEDICINE

Symptoms	Medicine
➣ Irregular periods. ➣ An acrid, watery vaginal discharge is experienced. ➣ A severe headache develops after the period has finished. ➣ Feelings of nervousness and tension.	◉ Natrum muriaticum
➣ Moody and changeable, cries a lot and also requires a lot of sympathy. ➣ Symptoms are much improved outdoors.	◉ Pulsatilla
➣ A sensation as if the contents of the pelvis are about to drop out. ➣ May feel cold, totally weary and tired, dislike their family, be irritable and feel very sad, but will liven up with exercise and movement.	◉ Sepia

Genital herpes

Genital herpes is caused by a virus. Women may find that bathing the lesions with a Hypericum and Calendula solution (five drops of mother tincture in about 290ml/½ pint of boiled and cooled water) provides some relief from the symptoms. Constitutional treatment may also be some help in preventing recurrences of the virus.

SYMPTOMS / MEDICINE

Symptoms	Medicine
➣ Burning stinging pain is relieved by cold applications. ➣ Pinkish local swelling (similar to the swelling around a bee sting) occurs.	◉ Apis mellifica
➣ Burning pain is much relieved by warm applications. ➣ A feeling of restlessness is present.	◉ Arsenicum album
➣ Sensitive lesions that feel hot and bleed easily.	◉ Borax
➣ Unbearable itching.	◉ Croton tiglium
➣ Vaginal dryness and lesions feel hot and look puffy.	◉ Natrum muriaticum
➣ Lesions on genitals, spreading to anus and thighs. ➣ Scratching tears skin which may become infected.	◉ Petroleum
➣ Genitals burn and itch. ➣ Symptoms are generally worse in cold, damp weather. ➣ A feeling of restlessness is present.	◉ Rhus toxicodendron

RHUS RADICANS
(R. TOXICODENDRON)

DOSAGE

USE THE 12C POTENCY. TAKE FOUR TIMES A DAY FOR FOUR DAYS.

Irritation of the genitalia

Pruritus vulvae

his type of irritation, which can become very severe and very distressing, is usually caused by, or is related to, a vaginal discharge (see page 30). It may also be present in those who are diabetic. The vaginal discharge that is experienced with the irritation can be caused by either an allergy to soaps or to other such bath products, or alternatively it can occur because the laundry detergent is not being completely rinsed out of the clothing during washing. Eczema may also be a cause of the vaginal irritation. *A vaginal discharge that causes irritation always requires medical diagnosis as soon as possible.*

SYMPTOMS / MEDICINE

Symptoms	Medicine
❧ Itching and pain apparent after intercourse. ❧ Nipples itch and burn. ❧ Bearing-down pains.	◉ Agaricus muscarius
❧ Itching with soreness and swelling. ❧ Bleeding occurs between periods (**consult your doctor**).	◉ Ambra grisea
❧ Itching, swelling and burning is present. ❧ An acrid vaginal discharge. ❧ Great fatigue accompanies periods.	◉ Ammonium carbonicum
❧ Burning and itching is present before and after the period, particularly in young girls.	◉ Calcarea carbonica
❧ Itching occurs at the vaginal orifice.	◉ Convallaria majalis
❧ Itching of the vulva and anus is accompanied by a bloody vaginal discharge.	◉ Copaiva officinalis
❧ Intense itching with pustular eruptions. ❧ Scratching is painful.	◉ Croton tiglium
❧ Itching and a yellow vaginal discharge occur and both seem worse when at rest. ❧ Elderly women are particularly prone.	◉ Fagopyrum esculentum
❧ Itching of the genitalia and nipples occurs during a period.	◉ Hepar sulphuris calcareum
❧ A burning itching within the vulva, with burning and swelling of the labia and violent itching between the labia and thighs.	◉ Kreosotum
❧ Swelling and intense itching of the vulva. ❧ Periods are early, profuse, prolonged and acrid, and cause vulval soreness.	◉ Rhus toxicodendron
❧ A yellow-green, irritating discharge is present. ❧ An intense bearing-down sensation in the pelvis.	◉ Sepia
❧ Vulva itches and the vagina burns because of an acrid, burning vaginal discharge.	◉ Sulphur

DOSAGE

USE THE 12C POTENCY TAKE THREE TIMES A DAY FOR FIVE DAYS.

Vaginal discharge

$\mathcal{M}$any women have a clear, non-irritating vaginal discharge, which is quite normal. *However, if the discharge becomes heavy or bloodstained, or if it causes burning or irritation, a doctor should always be consulted to determine the cause.* As most irritating discharges are sexually transmitted, both you and your partner must be treated. Conventional treatment, such as antibiotics and antifungals, is often necessary to rid the body of the causative organism. Apart from those produced by bacterial infections, the most common vaginal discharges are:

❧ **Candida or yeast infection**, which is caused by a yeast organism called *Candida albicans*. The symptoms are vaginal irritation, redness and swelling of the vulva and vagina, a cottage cheese-like discharge and often a burning sensation when passing urine.

❧ **Trichomonal infection (or Trich)** produces a frothy, smelly discharge with pain, irritation and soreness in the genital area and around the top of the thighs. Intercourse becomes painful and a burning sensation occurs when passing urine.

SYMPTOMS/MEDICINE

Symptoms	Medicine
❧ Very profuse, acrid, transparent or yellow discharge. ❧ Discharge occurs mainly during the daytime.	◉ Alumina
❧ Acrid, corrosive and yellow discharge. ❧ Discharge occurs mainly in the elderly and those with chronic diseases.	◉ Arsenicum album
❧ Clear, copious, hot discharge that is acrid. It causes swelling of the labia and is at its worst in mid-cycle.	◉ Borax
❧ Profuse, milky, itchy, burning discharge. ❧ Discharge present in young girls before puberty. ❧ Discharge occurs before the period in adults.	◉ Calcarea carbonica
❧ Discharge that is tenacious and thick. ❧ Weakness and constipation is also present.	◉ Hydrastis canadensis
❧ Profuse, thin, white mucous discharge which comes in gushes with associated back and lower abdominal pain. ❧ Discharge is more profuse in the morning on rising. ❧ Constantly cold.	◉ Graphites
❧ Profuse, watery, acrid, irritating and burning discharge, which causes soreness, smarting and itching of the vulva. ❧ Discharge is worse before a period.	◉ Kreosotum
❧ Yellow, stringy discharge is present in overweight, light-haired women.	◉ Kali bichromicum
❧ Watery, yellow-brown acrid discharge is present. ❧ Feelings of depression and a bearing-down sensation in the pelvis.	◉ Lilium tigrinum
❧ Acrid, burning, greenish-yellow discharge that causes smarting, burning and swelling of the vulva. ❧ Symptoms are worse at night.	◉ Mercurius solubilis
❧ Acrid, burning, creamy discharge accompanied by back pain.	◉ Pulsatilla
❧ Yellow-green offensive discharge. ❧ Discharge is worse before a period and there is a bearing-down sensation in the pelvis.	◉ Sepia
❧ Profuse, bland discharge of white mucus, accompanied by great weariness and backache.	◉ Stannum metallicum

DOSAGE

USE THE 30C POTENCY. TAKE TWICE A DAY FOR TEN DAYS.

Vaginismus

*T*he involuntary and painful spasm of the muscles of the vagina is known as vaginismus. Fortunately it is rare, but it does make sexual intercourse, the use of tampons and vaginal examination painful or impossible. Your doctor will probably suggest a gynecological referral if the cause is physical, but vaginismus is more likely to have a psychological cause, for which sex therapy is usually successful. While you are waiting, it is worth trying the medicines described here, but if they fail, you may need constitutional treatment.

SYMPTOMS / MEDICINE

Symptoms	Medicine
❧ Moods are changeable. ❧ Feels the cold but all the symptoms are relieved by warmth.	◉ Cimicifuga racemosa
❧ Vagina feels hot and burning. ❧ Feeling of restlessness. ❧ Intolerant of being touched, or of any movement.	◉ Belladonna
❧ If the vaginismus follows a broken love affair or grief.	◉ Ignatia amara
❧ Vaginismus resulting from great sensitivity of the vagina. ❧ Constipation is usually a problem.	◉ Plumbum metallicum
❧ Spasms of the vaginal muscles may be caused by anxiety. ❧ Painful intercourse followed by bleeding.	◉ Argentum nitricum
❧ Vagina feels as if it is grasped and held tightly. ❧ Intercourse is impossible.	◉ Cactus grandiflorus

DOSAGE

USE THE 30C POTENCY. TAKE TWICE A DAY FOR UP TO FIVE DAYS. REPEAT AS AND WHEN NECESSARY

Endometriosis

*E*ndometriosis is the name given to a condition in which small patches of cells similar to those that line the uterus (the endometrium) occur at other sites, such as on the ovaries, fallopian tubes, lower bowel and bladder. Very rarely, endometriosis can affect distant organs such as the eyes or lungs. The patches respond to the changing hormone levels of the menstrual cycle, and may shed blood at the time of the period causing local inflammation. If you have endometriosis you are likely to experience extremely painful periods.

The cause of endometriosis is unknown, but it may result from the menstrual flow spreading into the pelvis along the fallopian tubes and overwhelming the normal 'cleaning up' function of the body's immune system. You can boost your immune system by eating a good diet (see page 88). Orthodox treatment includes the use of hormone therapy and there are various surgical options. If you want to try homeopathy, you should consult a homeopath for constitutional treatment. (See also Painful periods, page 26.) ***Consult your doctor for investigation.***

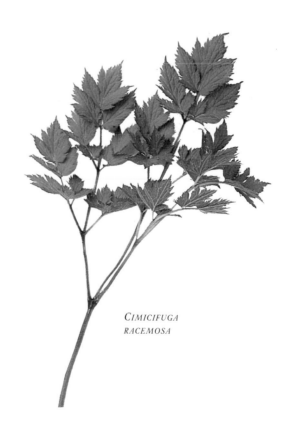

CIMICIFUGA RACEMOSA

CHAPTER 2

PREGNANCY, BIRTH & POST-PARTUM PROBLEMS

PRECONCEPTION CARE

In an ideal world preconception care would start at the time when a woman first has sex. Young people are being encouraged to use condoms to protect against AIDS, but for women another very important reason is for protection against the sexually transmitted infections that can result in infertility and increase the risk of ectopic (tubal) pregnancy.

If you are planning your first pregnancy, it is a good idea to start six months before the hoped-for date of conception. This will gives you time to ask your doctor to check if you are immune to rubella and to be immunized if necessary. It allows you to improve your diet (see The Food Triangle, page 88) and reduce, or preferably give up, smoking and alcohol (see pages 76–77 and page 119). Some doctors advise stopping the birth conception pill or having the coil taken out (if it contains copper) a couple of months before conception, to allow the reversal of the small changes these make to the body chemistry. During this time condoms or a diaphragm are the best methods of contraception. The ideal time to stop contraception, including the rhythm method, is immediately after a period, as this increases the likelihood of a freshly produced egg being fertilized by a recently deposited sperm, rather than either being past its best. Once pregnancy is confirmed, you should consult your doctor to decide where you wish to have your baby

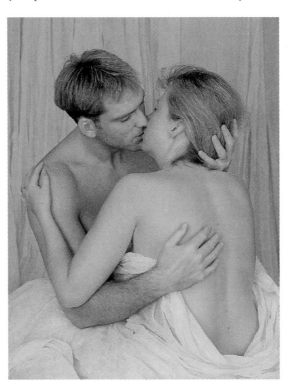

The ideal time to stop practising contraception with your partner is immediately after a period.

and to arrange prenatal care. Certain serious abnormalities, such as spina bifida and Down's syndrome, can now be diagnosed early enough in the pregnancy to allow you to consider a termination of the pregnancy. A rare but very serious complication is an ectopic pregnancy: that is, when the baby develops outside of the uterus. This is usually diagnosed between the sixth and tenth weeks of pregnancy, when it causes pain in the lower abdomen. It is essential to seek urgent medical advice if this condition is suspected.

PREGNANCY

The average human pregnancy lasts for about 38 weeks, but it is medical convention to date a pregnancy from the first day of the last period, so the delivery is expected to occur at 40 weeks. At the start of pregnancy the fertilized egg divides into cells that look identical but within a week the cells start to perform different functions. During the next few weeks the cells undergo special changes to become the baby's organs, such as the spinal cord and the heart. At the same time the placenta and membranes are formed. The placenta provides nourishment for the growing baby, and the membranes enclose the liquid that provides some protection from physical injury.

Until about 50 years ago doctors thought that the placenta was virtually an impregnable barrier, but it is now known that infections, such as rubella, and drugs, such as isotretinoin (thalidomide), can cross from mother to baby. Such environmental hazards are a particular problem during the first three months of pregnancy as this is when they can upset the delicate mechanisms that govern the formation of the organs.

For this reason, doctors are reluctant to prescribe any medication during the first three months of a pregnancy, unless the mother's life is at risk. This restriction includes mineral and vitamin supplements, apart from a small dose of folic acid. You should also avoid over-the-counter and herbal medicines, as well as social drugs, including illegal substances, alcohol and tobacco. There is no evidence that homeopathic medicines harm the baby in early pregnancy, but they should not be taken in potencies below 6c. They can be helpful for morning sickness, breast tenderness and other ailments that occur at this time.

Certain foods should be avoided during pregnancy. These include liver, which can contain large amounts of vitamin A, and soft cheeses and paté, which can contain listeria. Listeria is one cause of miscarriage and stillbirth, and unlike most bacteria it is able to grow at refrigerator temperature. It may also be present in pre-cooked and refrigerated foods, but these are safe if they are thoroughly heated before being eaten.

Toxoplasmosis infection can also seriously harm an unborn baby. If the expectant mother becomes infected, she may experience a mild fever, but may have no symptoms at all. In the United States the infection is uncommon, but, even so, pregnant women are advised to take steps to avoid the infection (see box).

In countries where toxoplasmosis is a common occurrence most women are immune to the disease because they have been infected before pregnancy. This can be confirmed by a blood test in early pregnancy. The few women who are susceptible are monitored during the pregnancy and treated accordingly if the infection is acquired.

LATER PREGNANCY

After the first three months of pregnancy there is a steady weight gain and the expectant mother likely to have put on 9–13 kg/20–28 lb by the time the baby is born. As the pregnancy progresses, most women feel fit

HOW TO AVOID TOXOPLASMOSIS

- ❧ Wash hands before preparing food and after handling raw meat or pets.
- ❧ Take care with raw meat: wash surfaces and utensils that have been in contact with it and do not let it contaminate other items that are in the refrigerator.
- ❧ Wash pet dishes separately from those used by the family.
- ❧ Cat litter trays should not be emptied by a pregnant woman.
- ❧ Wear gloves for gardening.

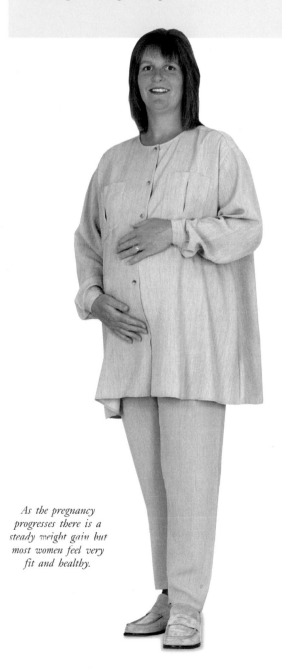

As the pregnancy progresses there is a steady weight gain but most women feel very fit and healthy.

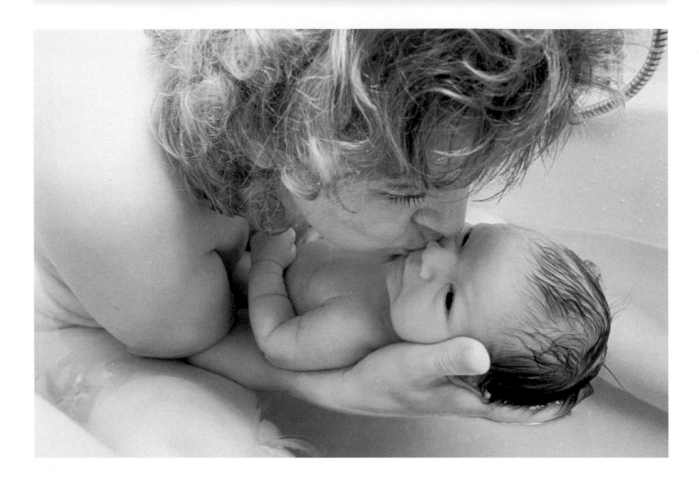

and healthy but others may develop annoying problems such as heartburn, constipation, backache and sleep problems. These will often respond very well to homeopathy without any danger to the pregnancy.

CHILDBIRTH

Doctors regard modern care during childbirth as a success because safety for both mother and baby has been greatly improved. Women, however, have been dismayed by the increased medical intervention in what they see as a 'natural' event. Fortunately, the tide is turning and there is now a wider choice about where to have their baby and whether to use underwater birthing and other non-orthodox approaches, including homeopathic medicines. Where these options are provided within the context of close medical supervision, safety is not compromised.

MISCARRIAGE

Two hundred years ago miscarriages were often welcomed by women whose frequent pregnancies were unregulated by effective contraception. Today with so much official advice on how to have a healthy baby, many women blame *You should have a choice about where to have your baby, and whether to use underwater birthing and other non-orthodox approaches, including homeopathic medicines.* themselves if they suffer a miscarriage, but they should not do so. The science of creating a healthy environment before birth is in its infancy and in practice it is not yet possible to be sure whether a miscarriage could have been prevented. For further information on miscarriage see page 35 and page 41.

STILLBIRTHS

Stillbirths can sometimes be explained, but all too often the cause remains a mystery and many women are unable to rid themselves of a sense of guilt and failure. Hospital staff are learning to provide more support and counseling after a stillbirth, but often it is the family, particularly the mother, who needs time and space to grieve. Homeopathy can help with both the physical and emotional problems of losing a pregnancy.

MISCARRIAGE

If you lose a pregnancy in the first six months, it is known as a miscarriage or spontaneous abortion; after this it is known as stillbirth. Between 10 and 30 per cent of pregnancies end in miscarriage, most frequently during the first three months.

CAUSES

- An abnormal foetus, such as a chromosomal abnormality or a major developmental defect.
- Hormonal deficiency.
- Fibroids or other deformity of the uterus.
- Failure of the cervix to remain closed (incompetent cervix).
- Maternal illness, such as high blood pressure, uncontrolled diabetes, infection or other serious illness.

SYMPTOMS

- Vaginal bleeding and/or cramping pain in the abdomen. In early pregnancy bleeding at the expected time of a period is quite common, as is bleeding from an erosion of the cervix.
- Backache.
- Disappearance of the symptoms of pregnancy, e.g. morning sickness.

WHAT YOU SHOULD DO

- Ring your doctor and go to bed.
- If you need to use a sanitary pad, do not flush it away as the doctor may want to examine it.

WHAT THE DOCTOR WILL RECOMMEND

- In early pregnancy your doctor is likely to recommend that you stay in bed and arrange for you to have an ultrasound scan. Doctors believe that a miscarriage during the first three months is usually the result of a serious foetal abnormality.
- In later pregnancy your doctor will probably refer you to a gynecologist because the likely causes, such as cervical incompetence, are often treatable.

AFTER THE MISCARRIAGE

- An ultrasound scan will show if the miscarriage has been complete: if not, you may need to be admitted to hospital for treatment to clear the uterus.

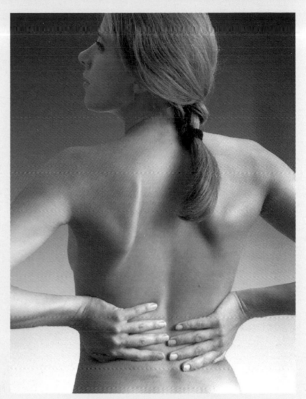

In early pregnancy, backache may be a symptom of a miscarriage.

- If your blood group is rhesus negative you should have a test for rhesus antibodies even after an early miscarriage. If these antibodies are present, you will require an injection to reduce the chance of damage to the baby in a later pregnancy.
- You will need to allow yourself time to grieve. If the miscarriage was a late one, and especially if you did not see the baby, do ask for a photograph.
- You can resume sexual intercourse when the bleeding has stopped and the cervix has closed. This is usually within a three week period. If you wish to try for another pregnancy straightaway, most doctors suggest that you wait for two normal menstrual periods after you have suffered an early miscarriage. Your doctor may suggest a longer wait after a late miscarriage, to allow your body to recover and to build up its stores of iron and calcium.
- The vast majority of women go on to have a normal pregnancy, but if you are unlucky enough to experience several miscarriages, your doctor will suggest tests to look for the cause.

Cramps and night cramps

A cramp is a prolonged, painful spasm in a muscle, most commonly due to either fatigue or imperfect posture. Cramps tend to be more frequent during pregnancy. Massaging the painful part is very helpful, but some pain, which feels like bruising, may be present for several hours after the cramp has been relieved.

SYMPTOMS/MEDICINE

Symptoms	Medicine
❧ Pain in soles of the feet. ❧ Tearing, painful contractions in the calves.	◉ Agaricus muscarius
❧ Cold, sweaty feet.	◉ Calcarea carbonica
❧ Pain occurs in the feet, which also feel numb if touched.	◉ Carbo vegetabilis
❧ Pain in the hip region and radiates to the knees. ❧ Cramp that is better for firm pressure and warmth.	◉ Colocynthis
❧ Cramp in calves and feet.	◉ Cuprum metallicum
❧ Cramp in forearm.	◉ Gelsemium sempervirens
❧ Arms and legs go to sleep. ❧ Cramp in the lower part of the legs. ❧ Arms and legs feel paralyzed in the morning.	◉ Nux vomica
❧ Cramp in neck and is relieved by warmth.	◉ Trifolium pratense
❧ Cramp in the calves. ❧ Skin feels cold. ❧ Fainting occurs from the least exertion.	◉ Veratrum album

DOSAGE

USE THE 12C POTENCY. TAKE AT BEDTIME AND WHEN CRAMP OCCURS.

Heavy legs

Y ou may experience a feeling of heaviness in your legs during the later stages of pregnancy. This may be due to your increased weight or to the fact that there is some pressure on the large veins that return the blood to the heart from the legs.

SYMPTOMS/MEDICINE

Symptoms	Medicine
❧ Legs feel heavy, weary and are difficult to move. ❧ Pressure is relieved by putting the feet up.	◉ Conium maculatum
❧ Trembling and weak legs are experienced. ❧ Fatigue after even the slightest exertion.	◉ Gelsemium sempervirens
❧ Red, bluish painful swelling of legs *(consult your doctor in case you have a blood clot)*. ❧ Legs are sensitive to the slightest touch.	◉ Lachesis mutus
❧ Heaviness, numbness and weakness of legs. ❧ Symptoms are worse for walking about. ❧ Legs are difficult to warm.	◉ Picricum acidum
❧ Legs feel dead or wooden. ❧ The symptoms are worst on first moving in the morning or just after rest. They improve with movement, but return when tired. ❧ A feeling of restlessness.	◉ Rhus toxicodendron

DOSAGE

USE THE 6C POTENCY. TAKE THREE TIMES A DAY FOR UP TO THREE WEEKS.

Swollen hands, ankles and feet

*I*f these symptoms occur, especially towards the end of pregnancy, your doctor or midwife should be consulted. In most cases they will be able to reassure you that the condition is due to simple causes, such as standing for too long, sitting for long periods in cramped conditions such as an airplane, your overall weight increase, or the pressure of the womb on the pelvic blood vessels. Sometimes, however, when the swelling is combined with raised blood pressure and the appearance of protein in the urine, it is a warning of pre-eclampsia. A homeopathic doctor will almost certainly prescribe constitutional treatment as well, *but this condition requires bed rest and conventional treatment, so consult your doctor.*

SYMPTOMS / MEDICINE

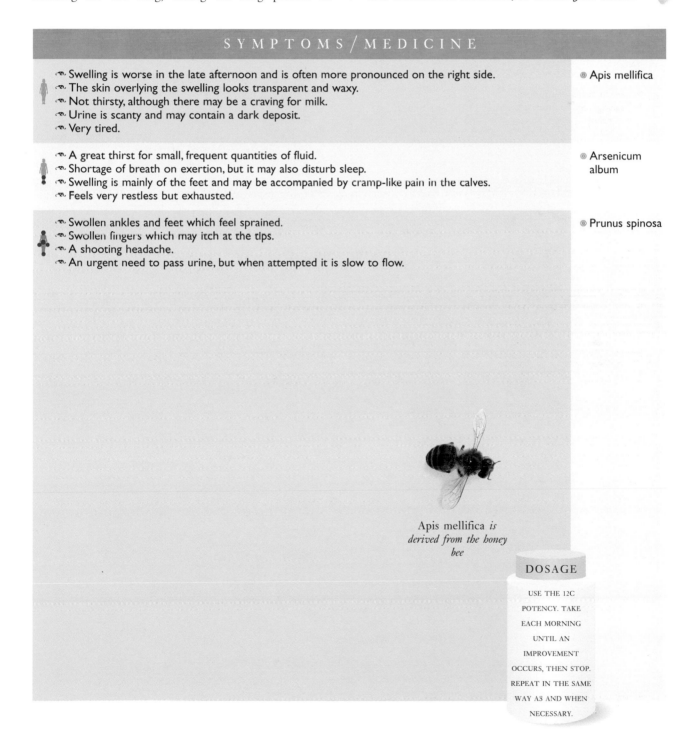

- Swelling is worse in the late afternoon and is often more pronounced on the right side.
- The skin overlying the swelling looks transparent and waxy.
- Not thirsty, although there may be a craving for milk.
- Urine is scanty and may contain a dark deposit.
- Very tired.

◉ Apis mellifica

- A great thirst for small, frequent quantities of fluid.
- Shortage of breath on exertion, but it may also disturb sleep.
- Swelling is mainly of the feet and may be accompanied by cramp-like pain in the calves.
- Feels very restless but exhausted.

◉ Arsenicum album

- Swollen ankles and feet which feel sprained.
- Swollen fingers which may itch at the tips.
- A shooting headache.
- An urgent need to pass urine, but when attempted it is slow to flow.

◉ Prunus spinosa

Apis mellifica *is derived from the honey bee*

DOSAGE

USE THE 12C POTENCY. TAKE EACH MORNING UNTIL AN IMPROVEMENT OCCURS, THEN STOP. REPEAT IN THE SAME WAY AS AND WHEN NECESSARY.

Cravings

Unusual, and sometimes bizarre, desires for certain foods may develop in pregnant women. These may be for unusual combinations of food or even, on some occasions, for indigestible substances like coal.

DOSAGE

USE THE 12C POTENCY. TAKE TWICE A DAY UNTIL THE CRAVING GOES.

SYMPTOMS / MEDICINE

Symptom	Medicine
A craving for meat, pickles, radishes, turnips, artichokes and coarse foods.	Abies canadensis
A craving for any food at noon and at night.	Abies nigra
An urgent need to eat sweets frequently.	Alfalfa
A craving for coffee.	Angustura vera
A craving for milk.	Apis mellifica
A craving for sweets.	Argentum nitricum
A craving for tobacco.	Caladium seguinum
A craving for indigestible things such as chalk and coal, as well as eggs, salt and sweets.	Calcarea carbonica
A craving for bacon, ham, salted meats and smoked meats.	Calcarea phosphorica
A craving for stimulants, including coffee, alcohol and tobacco.	Capsicum annuum
A craving for salt and salty foods.	Carbo vegetabilis
A craving for sweets.	Cina
A craving for anything and everything but the smell of it then nauseates.	Colchicum autumnale
A craving for sour and strongly flavored food.	Hepar sulphuris calcareum
A craving for wine.	Hypericum perforatum
A craving for some acidic foods.	Ignatia amara
A craving for alcohol and oysters.	Lachesis mutus
A craving for chocolate and sweet things.	Lycopodium clavatum
A craving for meat.	Magnesia carbonica
A craving for salt.	Natrum muriaticum
A craving for highly seasoned foods.	Nux moschata
A craving for ice water and as well as frequent glasses of cold drinks.	Onosmodium virginianum
A craving for all kinds of savory foods.	Sanguinaria canadensis
A craving for pickles and sour food and drink.	Sepia
A craving for cups of hot water.	Spigelia anthelmia
A craving for sweet and fatty foods.	Sulphur
A craving for apples.	Tellurium metallicum

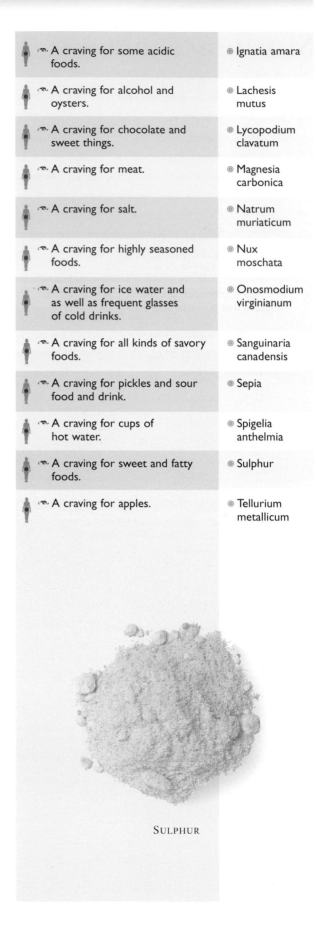

SULPHUR

Morning sickness

*V*omiting can be an irritating problem during early pregnancy. It is present in about half of pregnant women and it is most likely to occur with the first pregnancy. The severity is variable and usually amounts to a feeling of nausea on waking followed by a single episode of vomiting after getting out of bed, although the vomiting and nausea may occur at other times of the day. It usually starts during the second month and normally goes away by the end of the third month, although it can continue throughout the pregnancy. Although unpleasant, morning sickness does not normally affect your health. ***If the condition persists, or becomes excessive, a doctor should be consulted.***

SYMPTOMS / MEDICINE

Symptoms	Medicine
❧ Sour belching with heartburn. ❧ Profuse salivation day and night.	◉ Aceticum acidum
❧ Nausea is constantly present or comes in waves. ❧ Nausea that is worse after eating.	◉ Asarum europaeum
❧ Constant nausea which vomiting does not relieve. ❧ Despite vomiting, tongue remains clean, but excessive salivation may develop. ❧ A disinclination to eat. ❧ An irritable attitude.	◉ Ipecacuanha
❧ Continuous vomiting and unrelated to eating. ❧ The vomit tastes very acidic and bitter.	◉ Lac defloratum
❧ Nausea and there is a sour taste after breakfast. ❧ Stomach is very sensitive to pressure. ❧ May feel irritable and critical. ❧ Sensitivity to noise and smells. ❧ Much gas.	◉ Nux vomica
❧ Persistent and troublesome vomiting. ❧ Suits those who are anxious and nervous. ❧ A craving for cold drinks but these are vomited back. ❧ Vomiting may be precipitated by putting hands in hot water.	◉ Phosphorus
❧ Nausea at the sight or smell of food, especially in the morning before eating. ❧ Eating may temporarily relieve the nausea. ❧ A craving for sour foods. ❧ Stomach feels empty, even just after eating.	◉ Sepia

DOSAGE

USE THE 6C POTENCY. TAKE THREE TIMES A DAY UNTIL AN IMPROVEMENT OCCURS, THEN STOP. REPEAT IN THE SAME WAY AS AND WHEN NECESSARY.

Sleep problems

People who suffer from insomnia usually have difficulty only in falling asleep. Once asleep, most have no problem in remaining asleep. Difficulty in sleeping frequently occurs during pregnancy, especially in the final months. In the majority of women this is easily overcome with the use of a suitable relaxation technique and the correct homeopathic medicine, which will be safe to take in pregnancy and gives no risk of addiction or dependence. Insomnia of a different kind may, however, be present. With this kind, the woman wakes in the early morning (around 4–5 am) and this is then followed by short periods of unrefreshing sleep until it is time to get up. This type of sleeplessness can sometimes indicate the development of a depressive disorder and requires medical advice. It should not, however, be confused with another type of sleep disorder in which a woman is a very light sleeper, waking up with every slight noise but then immediately falling back to sleep again.

SYMPTOMS / MEDICINE

Symptoms	Medicine
Inability to fall asleep because of overexcitement during the evening. / Sleeplessness occurs because of fear.	Aconitum napellus
Insomnia caused by worry about an event the next day such as an examination or interview.	Argentum nitricum
An inability to fall asleep, or wakes up about 2 am. / Feels very restless and has to get up and walk around the room.	Arsenicum album
The problems of the day seem to go around and around in head. / Exciting thoughts of recent events causes wakefulness. / Great sensitivity to noise.	Coffea cruda
Sleeplessness associated with an unhappy or distressing event.	Ignatia amara
Wakes at about 4 am and cannot get back to sleep due to an overactive mind.	Lycopodium clavatum
Mental overactivity with the mind going over the day's work again and again. / Anger at the inability to fall asleep.	Nux vomica
Light sleepers are easily disturbed by the slightest noise.	Sulphur
Body feels itchy and there may be jerking movements of the limbs when attempting to fall asleep. / Unpleasant dreams often occur.	Valeriana officinalis

DOSAGE

USE THE 30C POTENCY. TAKE DURING THE EVENING IF POSSIBLE AND REPEAT AT BEDTIME. ANOTHER DOSE MAY BE TAKEN DURING THE NIGHT, IF NECESSARY.

Miscarriage
Spontaneous abortion

The ending of a pregnancy at an early stage with the loss of the fetus most frequently occurs during the first three months of a pregnancy and tends to start at the time when a period would have been due. Bleeding and regularly occurring lower abdominal pains are the usual early symptoms, and these become more pronounced until the pregnancy is expelled. Not all miscarriages are complete, and on occasions some tissue may be left in the uterus (womb) requiring a small operation under a general anesthetic to remove it. As not all threatened miscarriages result in loss of the pregnancy, absolute rest should always be part of the treatment. *Expert medical help should be sought as soon as a miscarriage is suspected. (See also box on page 35.)*

(See also box on page 35.)

DOSAGE

USE THE 30C POTENCY. IN THREATENED MISCARRIAGE TAKE FOUR TIMES A DAY UNTIL THE SYMPTOMS CEASE. AS A PREVENTIVE IN THOSE WITH A PREVIOUS HISTORY OF MISCARRIAGE, TAKE THREE TIMES A DAY ON THE SAME DAY OF EACH WEEK UNTIL THE 16TH WEEK.

SYMPTOMS / MEDICINE

Symptoms	Medicine
❧ Threatened miscarriage after anger.	◉ Aconitum napellus
❧ Threatened miscarriage after trauma.	◉ Arnica montana
❧ Profuse and hot-feeling bleeding with backache and headache. ❧ Labor-like pains come and go suddenly and there is a sensation as if everything is going to drop out of the pelvis.	◉ Belladonna
❧ Recurrent miscarriage. ❧ Severe pain develops in the back and sides of the abdomen and there also are feeble uterine contractions with a scanty blood loss.	◉ Caulophyllum thalictroides
❧ Anger with great agitation accompanies the miscarriage.	◉ Chamomilla
❧ Pains go from side to side across the lower part of the abdomen and causes doubling up. ❧ Helps those with a tendency to develop rheumatism.	◉ Cimicifuga racemosa
❧ Miscarriage occurs around the third month; bleeding is the first symptom, then pain develops in the small of the back and goes around and through to the front of the abdomen. ❧ The blood is bright red and clotted.	◉ Sabina
❧ Miscarriage occurs in very early pregnancy. ❧ Often suits those who are pale and in poor health. ❧ Frequent labor-like pains with a copious flow of very dark blood.	◉ Secale cornutum
❧ A preventive of miscarriage. ❧ Tendency to be nervous and irritable, accompanied by lax abdominal muscles and a tendency to rectal prolapse.	◉ Sepia
❧ Pain starts in the back, goes round to the front of the abdomen, then down into the thighs. ❧ Used in frequent and early miscarriages.	◉ Viburnum opulus

After miscarriage

The main problem following a miscarriage is usually emotional, as the experience can be mentally traumatic. The advice given for anxiety, depression and grief (see pages 124, 126 and 128) will help in dealing with this. The other main problem is that the periods, when they restart, may be rather erratic. Treatment for this can be found on page 25.

DOSAGE

USE THE 30C POTENCY. TAKE FOUR TIMES A DAY FOR FOUR DAYS.

SYMPTOMS / MEDICINE	
➤ Low back pain with prolapse. ➤ Periods either stop or become very heavy and frequent.	⊚ Helonias dioica
➤ Backache with excessive tiredness.	⊚ Kali carbonicum
➤ Profuse periods of bright red, partly clotted blood.	⊚ Ustilago maidis

Ectopic pregnancy

An ectopic pregnancy is one that occurs outside the uterus, (womb), usually in one of the fallopian tubes. As the narrow tube is unable to expand to accommodate the growing fetus, it will eventually rupture, usually between the sixth and tenth weeks, causing pain in the lower part of the abdomen. Haemorrhage can be severe and an ectopic pregnancy is a medical emergency. *If you suspect an ectopic pregnancy, you should contact your doctor or midwife at once.* An ectopic pregnancy is usually removed surgically, and although the gynecologist will endeavor to preserve the fallopian tube, this is often not possible. Afterwards you may experience physical and emotional problems similar to those following a miscarriage (see page 41 and left). If you are anxious and apprehensive while waiting for medical attention, take Aconitum.

DOSAGE

USE THE 30C POTENCY. TAKE EVERY THIRTY MINUTES UNTIL YOU FEEL BETTER.

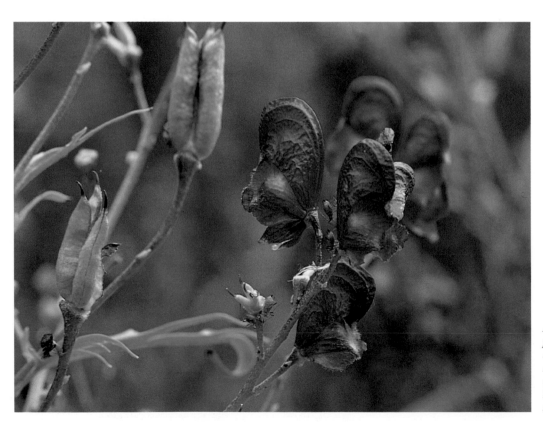

Aconitum, which is prepared from the deadly poisonous plant, Aconitum napellus, calms the deep fears that lead to anxiety, panic and frantic impatience.

False labor

*L*abor-like contractions may occur in the last few weeks of pregnancy and are felt irregularly, usually in the lower part of the abdomen. These are said to occur because the uterus (womb) is 'toning-up' in preparation for the birth of the baby. *If the contractions become very frequent or regular, or if there is a 'show' of blood, the doctor or midwife should be called.*

SYMPTOMS / MEDICINE

Symptoms	Medicine
◠ Contractions that occur early in the pregnancy. ◠ Pain shoots across the abdomen, causing doubling up.	◉ Cimicifuga racemosa
◠ Contractions that occur in the last few weeks of pregnancy.	◉ Caulophyllum thalictroides
◠ Pain goes up the back and into the hips.	◉ Gelsemium sempervirens
◠ Colicky, cramp-like pains.	◉ Viburnum opulus

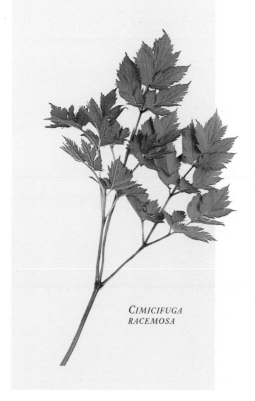

CIMICIFUGA RACEMOSA

Preparing for delivery

*F*or most women homeopathic medicine can help enormously in the run up to birth of a baby. By taking Caulophyllum in the last weeks of the pregnancy and Arnica before delivery, much of the bruising and bleeding that occurs will be minimized. Caulophyllum is also said to 'tone up' the uterus, helping to produce good contractions and lessening the chances of the mother becoming overtired during labor.

SYMPTOMS / MEDICINE

Symptoms	Medicine
◠ Reduces the bruising and bleeding of normal labour	◉ Arnica montana
◠ Used routinely to help uterine contractions and to bring about a smooth delivery.	◉ Caulophyllum thalictroides
◠ May help if there was heavy bleeding in a previous pregnancy.	◉ Millefolium

In early labor

A normal pregnancy lasts for 40 weeks. For a few weeks before the birth occasional painless 'contractions' may be felt in the lower abdomen (see False labor, page 43). When you start labor proper, the contractions become noticeable but may be infrequent and irregular. As labor proceeds, they become more frequent and occur at regular intervals. They may also produce some discomfort. At first they are often felt in the back. The start of labor may be indicated by a small blood loss called a 'show'. At some stage the membranes in which the baby is contained will rupture, producing a loss of a watery fluid from the vagina. This is perfectly normal. The actual duration of labor varies tremendously, but is lengthier with a first pregnancy, so there is usually plenty of time in which to get to your hospital or for your midwife to arrive if you are having a home delivery.

SYMPTOMS / MEDICINE

Symptoms	Medicine
↝ When the labor pains are frequent but irregular. ↝ A good remedy if restless, anxious and frightened, and convinced of dying during labor.	⊛ Aconitum napellus
↝ Painful labor, with the pain starting in lower back and radiating to inner part of the thighs. ↝ May be overexcited and cross, and resents being examined. ↝ Intolerance of pain.	⊛ Chamomilla
↝ Spasmodic irregular pains in the small of the back. ↝ Feelings of exhaustion and being out of control.	⊛ Cocculus indicus
↝ Contractions are very painful but ineffective. ↝ Restless and agitated attitude.	⊛ Coffea cruda
↝ Intermittent, relatively painless contractions with little progress. ↝ Excessive tiredness.	⊛ Gossypium herbaceum
↝ Early labor pains in back.	⊛ Kali carbonicum

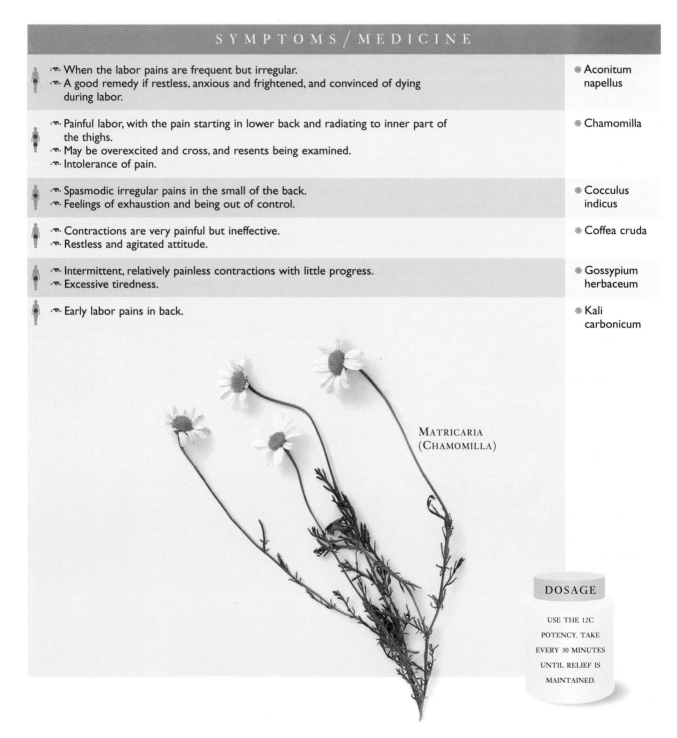

MATRICARIA
(CHAMOMILLA)

DOSAGE

USE THE 12C POTENCY. TAKE EVERY 30 MINUTES UNTIL RELIEF IS MAINTAINED.

Immediately after delivery

*T*he mother's main problems after the baby has been born will be related to the bruising that occurs in the birth passage and surrounding organs such as the bladder and urethra. With a prolonged labor, or one that has caused much sleep deprivation, fatigue can also be a

DOSAGE

USE THE 12C POTENCY. TAKE THREE TIMES A DAY FOR FIVE DAYS.

problem, but this is easily remedied by a good night's sleep. Following a birth by Caesarean section, the main problems tend to be those which any surgical procedure may produce. Most of these complications are unlikely to occur if you have been treated with Arnica and Caulophyllum, as described on page 43. The other group of after-delivery problems will relate to feeding the baby, and advice on how to treat these is on page 47. See also After-pains, page 46.

SYMPTOMS / MEDICINE

Symptoms	Medicine
❧ Difficulty passing urine. ❧ Restless, sleepless and frightened.	◉ Aconitum napellus
❧ Constipation. ❧ Rectum feels sore and anus itches. ❧ Even a soft stool is passed with difficulty.	◉ Alumina
❧ There are problems passing urine.	◉ Arsenicum album
❧ Irritation of the vulva. ❧ Cramp-like pains occur in the uterus (womb), mainly at night.	◉ Caladium seguinum
❧ Retention of urine, especially after a long labor.	◉ Causticum
❧ Nervousness and restlessness.	◉ Chamomilla
❧ Excited, oversensitive and suffers from insomnia. ❧ Abdominal pains.	◉ Coffea cruda
❧ Painful piles or hemorrhoids.	◉ Collinsonia canadensis
❧ Gas and abdominal colic.	◉ Nux moschata
❧ Back pain. ❧ Itching between the breasts. ❧ Apathy.	◉ Phosphoricum acidum
❧ Piles or hemorrhoids and anal prolapse occur.	◉ Podophyllum
❧ Total exhaustion and overheating.	◉ Secale cornutum
❧ To aid healing if there has been catheterization or an episiotomy.	◉ Staphysagria

CAUSTICUM

After-pains

These are pains similar to labor pains, that may occur after childbirth. They are a result of the uterus (womb) contracting as it reduces back to its previous size before the pregnancy occurred. The pains are more likely to happen if you are breast-feeding your baby as the action causes the pituitary gland to release a hormone called oxytocin, which helps with the milk production and may also stimulate some uterine contractions.

SYMPTOMS / MEDICINE

Symptoms	Medicine
Used routinely after all labors, especially if labor has been protracted.	Arnica montana
After-pains with a headache, flushed face, nervousness and restlessness.	Belladonna
Soreness felt all through the pelvis, making walking and standing painful. Legs feel as if they will give way.	Bellis perennis
Severe, cramp-like pains.	Camphora
Spasmodic pains occur which move across the lower abdomen, especially after a prolonged and exhausting labor. Quite specifically for after-pains.	Caulophyllum thalictroides
Severe pain causing great irritability.	Chamomilla
Intense pains like electric shocks in the groin. Agitated and intolerant of pain.	Cimicifuga racemosa
Pains which feel as if they are in the intestines rather than the uterus.	Cocculus indicus
Extreme pain causing sleeplessness.	Coffea cruda
Distressing after-pains after pregnancy that is not the first.	Cuprum metallicum
Anxious, apprehensive, sleepless.	Gelsemium sempervirens
Severe after-pains shoot down the thighs and are worse on the right. Pain appears to be in the rectum or the bladder.	Lac caninum
Large blood clots may be passed. Much gas.	Nux vomica
Pain shoots forwards from behind.	Sabina
Pain radiates upwards. A sensation of a weight in the lower bowel. Pelvic organs feel as though they are about to drop out.	Sepia
Use this if there are no other symptoms and no other homeopathic remedy seems to fit.	Xanthoxylum fraxineum

DOSAGE

USE THE 30C POTENCY. TAKE FOUR TIMES A DAY FOR TWO DAYS AFTER DELIVERY.

Engorgement

Engorgement is the overfilling of the breasts with milk. It is a common occurrence a few days after childbirth when the milk begins to be produced in quantity. Alternatively, it may occur if you need to stop breast-feeding suddenly for some reason. See Feeding difficulties, below, for medicines.

⅛

Feeding difficulties

Lactation is the time after birth when the mother secretes milk. Generally, lactation becomes well established, giving good-quality milk without too much trouble. In some cases, however, one of three things may happen: too much milk is produced, too little milk is produced, or the milk is of a poor quality and does not satisfy the baby. See also Sore and cracked nipples, page 48.

SYMPTOMS / MEDICINE

Symptoms	Medicine
↝ Too much milk is being produced and flows very freely. ↝ Breasts become red, hot, swollen and tender, and may be rock hard. ↝ Flushed and feels hot.	⊛ Belladonna
↝ A stitching pain in the breast just used for feeding.	⊛ Borax
↝ Much watery, poor-quality milk is produced, which the baby is reluctant to take. ↝ Chilly with feelings of anxiety and fear. ↝ Excessive perspiration during the night, mainly on the head.	⊛ Calcarea carbonica
↝ Milk production stops. ↝ Great depression, development of great thirst, and forecasts of own death occurring within the next 24 hours.	⊛ Lac defloratum
↝ Excess milk is produced, breasts feel hard, lumpy and painful, and nipples are intensely sensitive ↝ Body hurts all over and there is irritability and restlessness.	⊛ Phytolacca decandra
↝ The milk is thin and watery, and little is produced. ↝ Tendency to cry when trying to feed the baby. ↝ Breasts may feel sore and stretched. ↝ Milk continues to be produced after feeding has ceased.	⊛ Pulsatilla
↝ Painful distension of the breasts.	⊛ Rhus toxicodendron
↝ Little or no milk is being produced. ↝ Feelings of weakness in both mind and body.	⊛ Ricinus communis
↝ A much diminished flow of milk. ↝ Breasts become excessively swollen and tender.	⊛ Urtica urens

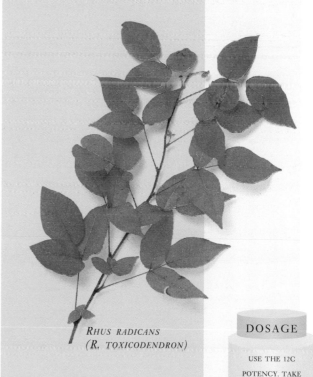

RHUS RADICANS (R. TOXICODENDRON)

DOSAGE

USE THE 12C POTENCY. TAKE TWICE A DAY UNTIL AN IMPROVEMENT OCCURS, THEN STOP. REPEAT AS AND WHEN NECESSARY.

Sore and cracked nipples

𝒯his is a frequent problem that occurs with mothers who are breast-feeding their babies. Local treatment to the nipple with Hypercal lotion (10 drops in 100ml/⅓ cup of cool boiled water four times a day) is helpful, and Calendula cream (applied three times a day) can be used to soften and soothe the sensitive nipple area. If the nipple becomes cracked, Graphites ointment (applied locally three times a day) may also be used to treat the breast in conjunction with the selected medicine from below.

SYMPTOMS / MEDICINE

Symptoms	Medicine
⤳ Soreness and itching.	⊛ Agaricus muscarius
⤳ Inflamed and very tender nipples. ⤳ Cannot bear the pain. ⤳ Very irritable.	⊛ Chamomilla
⤳ Nipples are very sore to touch and feeding is painful. ⤳ Pain goes around the chest wall to the back.	⊛ Croton tiglium
⤳ Cracks and soreness in the nipples. ⤳ Nipples bleed during feeding.	⊛ Lycopodium clavatum
⤳ Nipples are very sensitive with splinter-like pain. ⤳ Very chilly.	⊛ Nitricum acidum
⤳ Sore and cracked nipples, which are also very sore on feeding. ⤳ Breasts feel lumpy. ⤳ Pain seems to go all over the body, radiating from the breasts.	⊛ Phytolacca decandra
⤳ Extreme pain when feeding. ⤳ Very sensitive, emotional and bad tempered. ⤳ The least word can cause an upset.	⊛ Staphysagria
⤳ Nipples smart and burn after feeding.	⊛ Sulphur

DOSAGE

USE THE 30C POTENCY. TAKE THREE TIMES A DAY FOR THREE DAYS.

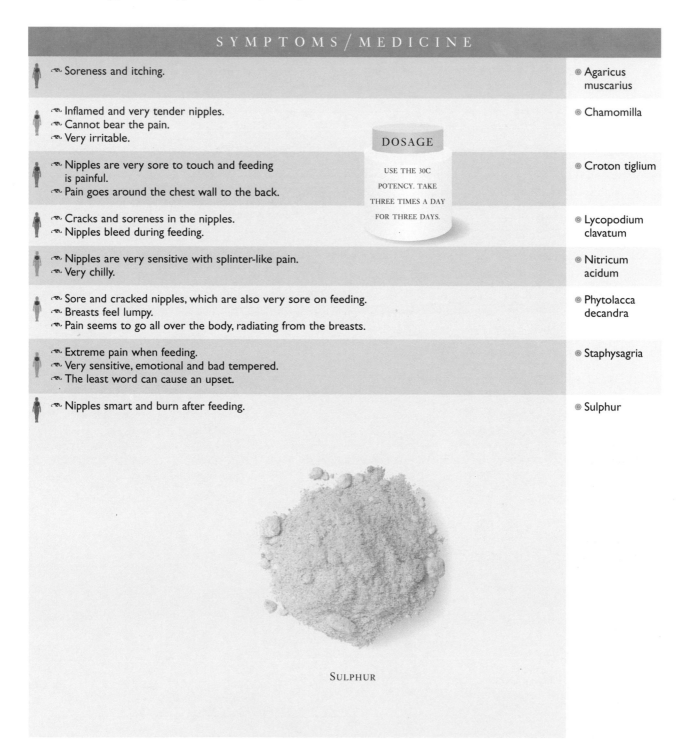

SULPHUR

Post-partum depression

*C*ommonly known as post-partum 'blues', many new mothers experience post-partum depression in a very mild form for a few days, usually when they return home from the hospital and have to face the responsibility of looking after the new baby plus the rest of the family and their home. Occasionally, however, a much more serious and dangerous form of depression occurs. *This requires skilled medical care to cure and a doctor should be consulted about it as soon as the symptoms first become apparent.*

SYMPTOMS / MEDICINE

Symptoms	Medicine
• Mental restlessness with great fear, especially of death, worst between midnight and 3 am. • May feel suicidal and want to refuse treatment that is felt to be useless.	⊛ Arsenicum album
• Feelings of unworthiness, but quarrelsome, contradictory and oversensitive to noise. • Moans in sleep and may wake at 4 am, then only able to catnap.	⊛ Aurum metallicum
• Sad and hopeless, the slightest comment causes weeping and the slightest criticism leads to anger. • Mental exhaustion with frequent and rapid mood changes. • Feels that will never again be able to sleep properly. • Depression follows grief, loss of sleep and sudden emotional situations. • Nervous and sensitive, easily excited and easily offended. • Full of contradictions, such as laughing at sad news.	⊛ Ignatia amara
• Desires and is helped by sympathy. • Soothed by being touched and stroked. • Full of fear about virtually anything. • Feels worse lying on left side. • Oversensitive to light, noise and smells. • A thirst for cold drinks, which are often vomited back after reaching the stomach. • Suited to those who are tall and slender with fine hair and long eyelashes.	⊛ Phosphorus
• Needs a lot of sympathy. • Restless, especially at night, and often gets up to wander around the house. • Sad and cries easily, especially when feeding the baby. • A tendency to burst into tears when talking about own problems, but the sadness quickly passes when consoled. • Changeable, contradictory moods. • Feels much better outdoors and when moving about gently. • May shiver easily even though dislikes the heat. • A preference for cold food, and a lack of thirst despite a dry mouth.	⊛ Pulsatilla
• Feels indifferent to the baby, husband and family and feels the need to get away, but dreads being alone • Hates sympathy, which when given, leads to tears. • Feels better for eating, but becomes nauseous at the smell of cooking. • Easily offended. • Feels physically and mentally exhausted.	⊛ Sepia

DOSAGE

USE THE 30C POTENCY. TAKE THREE TIMES A DAY FOR FOUR OR FIVE DAYS

CHAPTER 3

THE MENOPAUSE

HE WORD MENOPAUSE literally means the cessation of the monthly periods and in most women it occurs around the age of 50. However, the final period is only one of a number of events that occur around this time of life, which is frequently called 'the change' or 'change of life'. These are excellent descriptions as there are many changes that occur as a result of decreased hormone levels. The medical term is the 'climacteric'.

PERIODS AND FERTILITY

Most women notice changes in their menstrual cycles some time after the age of about 40. First the length of the cycle often shortens, by as much as ten days, then it becomes longer and eventually the periods cease. Sudden cessation of periods is unusual.

Ovulation does not occur with every cycle in the forties and thus fertility drops rapidly at this time. However, doctors advise that you should continue to use contraception until either a year after the last period, or until hormone levels suggest that menopause has occurred. You should consult your doctor about very heavy, painful periods and also bleeding between periods as these are not necessarily caused by the change. Bleeding that occurs more than a year after your last period also needs to be investigated.

BODY CHANGES

Decreased hormonal levels cause a number of physical changes. The most obvious are hot flushes and night sweats, vaginal dryness and, for some women, painful joints. Also the risk of angina and heart attacks increases, and the bones lose calcium more quickly.

As the change progresses, the tissues under the skin become flabbier, and loss of tone in the pelvic muscles can lead to prolapse and stress incontinence. Homeopathic symptom medicines for many of these conditions are suggested in this chapter, but constitutional help may also be needed.

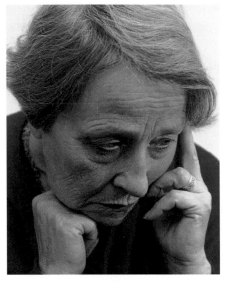

Many women feel secretly, or openly, unhappy about changes in their looks which can occur around the menopause.

HORMONE REPLACEMENT THERAPY (HRT)

Your doctor may suggest using HRT, which often eases the symptoms that occur during the change. However, HRT does not suit or even help every woman, and if personal preference or medical reasons dictate that it should not be used, then homeopathy can offer considerable help in smoothing the change for the woman from the reproductive to non-reproductive state. The decision is obviously a complex one and it is wise to discuss the whole matter with your doctor who may consider prescribing estrogen cream for vaginal dryness, if this is an isolated problem that is not helped by using a lubricating cream, such as KY jelly.

MENTAL SYMPTOMS

Falling estrogen levels may cause mild anxiety or depression and these can cause great concern, but you may be reassured to know that serious depressive illness is no more likely during the change than at other times of life. However, other events, such as the so-called 'empty nest syndrome' when the children leave home, or the death or increasing dependence of elderly relatives, often occur at around the same time and may cause some psychological stress. During the change, some women experience a lack of interest in sex and an inability to reach orgasm, whether or not they also experience vaginal dryness. Others may experience a greatly increased sex drive and this may lead them to seek extra-marital relationships.

Many women feel secretly, or openly, unhappy about the changes in their looks, sometimes made worse by the onset of skin problems such as dryness or acne rosacea, and occasionally they lose interest in their personal appearance, their work and the home. All these factors can lead to diminished self-esteem, job loss and even possible marital break-up. Many of these psychological difficulties respond well to homeopathy but constitutional treatment may be required, so if you are not helped by the medicines suggested in either this section or the section on emotional problems, it is well worth consulting a homeopath.

After the menopause

Today, many more women can look forward to 30 or more years of life after menopause. You may not be able to take good health for granted in quite the same way as you once could, but there is much you can do to help you live these years to the full.

DIET

Attention to diet remains of continuing importance. There is increasing evidence that older people need a high-quality diet, with at least the full five portions-a-day of fruit and vegetables, to boost their immune system in its fight against infection and cancer (see page 88). Recent research also suggests that dark green leafy vegetables may help to prevent some of the more common causes of blindness. If your teeth object to chewing fruit and vegetables, use a blender.

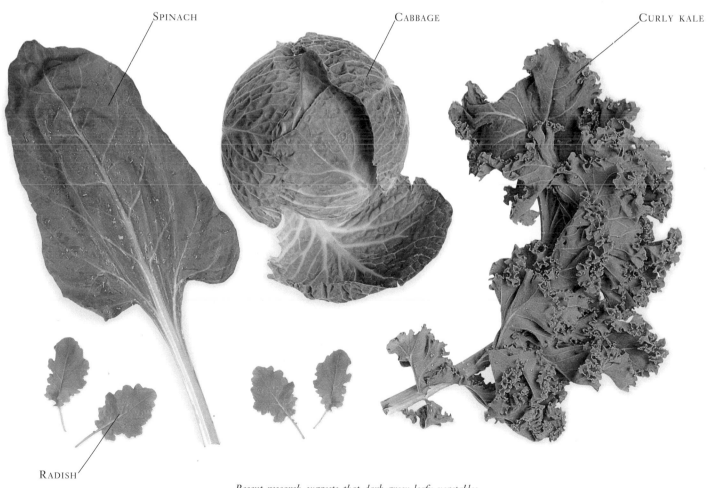

SPINACH

CABBAGE

CURLY KALE

RADISH

Recent research suggests that dark green leafy vegetables may help to prevent blindness in older people.

WEIGHT

Older people require fewer calories daily since they tend to be less active and more easily put on weight. Being overweight aggravates a number of medical conditions, such as diabetes and high blood pressure, and leads to greater wear and tear of arthritic joints. Very strict diets should be avoided (unless under medical supervision), and it is best to concentrate on healthy eating. Regular exercise is also helpful, especially swimming as this does not stress the joints too much. Many swimming pools cater for older users by allocating them a special time.

DIABETES

Some older people may develop diabetes. It produces few symptoms and is often found when your doctor makes a routine check of your urine, or your optician notices changes in the retina at the back of your eyes. If your parents or grandparents developed old-age diabetes, ask your doctor to check your urine from time to time, especially if you are overweight.

Old-age diabetes rarely requires insulin and your doctor will usually suggest dietary changes and medication. There are some homeopathic medicines that can be helpful, but these should not be introduced without medical supervision.

OSTEOPOROSIS

The density of bones decreases in older people, and is particularly marked in women after the menopause. Osteoporosis is a serious condition, as thin bones will break easily. The standard medical treatment is to recommend HRT, but about 80 per cent of women cannot, or do not wish to, use it. If you are one of them, you can adopt other measures to decrease your risk of osteoporosis (see box on right).

CARING FOR THE AGED

More and more people are living to old age, and much of their care is provided by their families. If you are a care giver, do not be afraid to give the homeopathic symptom medicines described in this book. They provide a very gentle treatment and do not interfere with other medication that has been prescribed.

OSTEOPOROSIS

Hormone replacement therapy is not the only way to preserve the strength of your bones. It is never too late to start keeping your bones strong by adopting the following suggestions.

CHANGE YOUR DIET

- Consume 1000–1500mg of calcium a day (see food list, right). Do not exceed 2000mg.
- Eat plenty of green, yellow and red vegetables, and fruit.
- Do not eat too much protein.

CUT DOWN ON . . .

- Alcohol (three drinks a day maximum).
- Caffeine (in coffee, tea, cola and many over-the-counter painkillers).
- Salt.

TAKE PLENTY OF EXERCISE

Take at least 30 minutes three times a week (see suggestions list on page 53), if you are up and about. If not, do move about as much as you possibly can.

SUNLIGHT

Expose your skin to outdoor sunlight on as many days as possible. Try to allow the sun on your skin (without sunblock) for 15 to 30 minutes before 10 am or during the late afternoon, when the sun is less strong. Save time by taking your exercise outside.

SMOKING

Stop smoking (see page 85) and avoid illegal drugs.

MEDICINES

AVOID THE FOLLOWING OVER-THE-COUNTER MEDICINES . . .

- Laxatives: instead, gradually increase the fiber in your diet and reduce the dose.
- Antacids that contain aluminum: if you have to take antacids, use those containing calcium instead.

SOME FOODS HIGH IN CALCIUM

food	amount	approximate mg of calcium
Skimmed milk	150ml/5 fl oz	180
Natural yoghurt	100g/4oz	180
Cheddar cheese	50g/2oz	400
Canned salmon, plus bones	100g/4oz	195
Canned sardines, plus bones	100g/4oz	460
Dried figs	100g/4oz	280
Red kidney beans, cooked	100g/4oz	140
Almonds	100g/4oz	250
Molasses	25g/1oz	170
Raw celery	100g/4oz	50
Broccoli	100g/4oz	75
Raw parsley	25g/1oz	80
Watercress	50g/2oz	110
Tap water, soft	1 litre/1¾ pints	10–30
Tap water, hard	1 litre/1¾ pints	100

EXERCISE SUGGESTIONS

Vary your exercise regime to avoid getting bored and to benefit different bones. Don't forget to warm up properly first. If you have any health problems, always check with your doctor before you start any exercise programme.

❧ Walking benefits your feet, legs, hips and lower back. Walk fast enough to be a little out of breath but still able to talk.

❧ Running and dancing help the same bones, but are tougher on weight-bearing joints that are affected by early arthritis.

❧ Tennis benefits the same bones, plus the upper back and also the wrists.

❧ Cycling, golf, rowing (boat or machine), windsurfing and bowling (indoor or outdoor) all benefit the bones of the arms and legs.

❧ Weight training doesn't have to be done in a gym: use cans and plastic bottles from your store cupboard to strengthen bones in your arms and upper back.

❧ Yoga is probably best learned in a class that is taught by an experienced instructor. Choose a group that matches your age.

Yoga can be very beneficial to your body as you get older as it will help you to breathe properly and keep you toned and very supple.

Absent-mindedness
Poor memory

The symptoms outlined below occur in addition to the absent-mindedness.

SYMPTOMS/MEDICINE	
• Nervous indigestion is noticed. • Depression and irritability is felt. • A decreased sense of smell, sight and hearing.	⊛ Anacardium orientale
• A weak memory becomes apparent.	⊛ Argentum nitricum
• Feelings of apathy and lifelessness.	⊛ Aurum metallicum
• There is debility and hypochondriasis. • Poor memory is accompanied by disorders of the urinary tract and sexual weakness.	⊛ Conium maculatum
• Incoherent conversation with silly and nonsensical behavior.	⊛ Duboisisa myoporoides
• There is impaired coordination. • Numbness and tingling in the limbs.	⊛ Kali bromatum
• Memory is weak. • Confused thoughts. • Mistakes are made when writing and spelling.	⊛ Lycopodium clavatum
• Loss of will-power. • Weak memory	⊛ Mercurius solubilis
• Confusion and an impaired memory.	⊛ Nux moschata
• Slow perception. • Memory is weak.	⊛ Oleander
• Dizziness and a feeling of haziness. • An urge to talk continuously.	⊛ Physalis alkekengi

DOSAGE

USE THE 12C
POTENCY.
TAKE TWICE A DAY
UNTIL AN
IMPROVEMENT IS
MAINTAINED.

Sleep disturbances

An inability to sleep well is a frequent trial of the menopause. Commonly, women find it difficult to fall asleep and then to remain asleep. This is a time when it is therefore very easy to get into the habit of taking conventional sleeping pills. Unfortunately, this is not the best thing to do as dependence is quickly established and the dosage may need to be steadily increased to guarantee sleep.

Homeopathic remedies, which are available from most homeopathic pharmacies, offer a safe, gentle, non-addictive alternative with no risk of a 'hung over' feeling in the morning. More information about specific medicines for sleep problems is given in the Pregnancy section, page 40.

There are also some self-help methods you can try to help you get to sleep:

1 Relax before going to bed: read a book, have a warm bath, make love.
2 Avoid large meals late in the evening.
3 Take a bedtime drink of warm milk or a herbal tea, but avoid drinking tea, coffee or chocolate drinks that contain caffeine.
4 Extra exercise earlier in the day will make you more tired physically.
5 If you wake in the night don't toss and turn, get up and do something for half an hour.
6 Get up at the same time every day even if you have had a bad night.

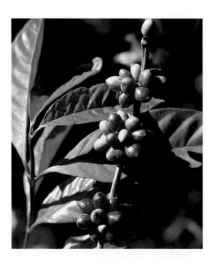

If you are finding it difficult to sleep during the menopause, Coffea cruda is a non-addictive homeopathic medicine that can be helpful.

Acne rosacea

Acne rosacea is a skin complaint that appears on the flush areas on the cheeks. It develops particularly in women at the menopause. The small blood vessels near the skin surface dilate and the sebaceous follicles increase in size. Rosacea is often complicated by an acne-type eruption. Excessive tea-drinking is often associated with this complaint, as are oranges, orange juice and chocolate.

SYMPTOMS / MEDICINE

Symptoms	Medicine
Rosacea with violet pimples on the nose. Worse in the spring.	Arsenicum bromatum
Skin feels dry and hot but may alternate between redness and being pale.	Belladonna
Rash is more copper-colored than red.	Carbo animalis
A purple rash that is worse for warmth.	Kali iodatum
A yellow-brownish rash involving the cheeks and nose in a saddle-like distribution is apparent.	Sepia
Scanty periods and poor circulation. Hot flushes and red cheeks that are both worse for warmth.	Sanguinaria canadensis
A rash on the tip of the nose as well as the cheeks.	Causticum
Small, red pimples on the face.	Psorinum

DOSAGE

USE THE 6C POTENCY. TAKE TWICE A DAY UNTIL AN IMPROVEMENT OCCURS, THEN STOP. REPEAT IN THE SAME WAY AS AND WHEN NECESSARY.

Fibroids

Fibroids are non cancerous tumors lying either in the walls of the uterus or on its surface. They are very common after the age of 35 but often disappear naturally after about 45. If your fibroids are small you may not experience any symptoms but they are a cause of heavy, sometimes painful, periods. Occasionally they grow large enough to interfere with the normal activities of the bladder and bowel. They may be the reason for failure to conceive or recurrent miscarriages. Conventional treatment is surgical; homeopathic treatment is usually constitutional, but you may find the following medicines helpful. *You should consult your doctor if bleeding occurs between your periods.*

DOSAGE

USE THE 12C POTENCY. TAKE TWICE A DAY UNTIL AN IMPROVEMENT OCCURS, THEN STOP. REPEAT AS AND WHEN NECESSARY.

SYMPTOMS / MEDICINE

Symptoms	Medicine
Uterus is enlarged and may be painful. Vaginal spasms and a constant vaginal discharge.	Aurum muriaticum
There are small fibroids with a yellow vaginal discharge. May experience period pains before the period starts.	Calcarea iodata
Short painful periods and an intolerance of clothing or covers. Symptoms are relieved as the period starts. A remedy that is particularly useful at the menopause.	Lachesis
Large fibroids. Periods are heavy, painful and occur early. Restlessness.	Tarentula hispana

Hot sweats and flushes

*F*lushes and sweats are possibly the most common and certainly among the most distressing features of the menopause.

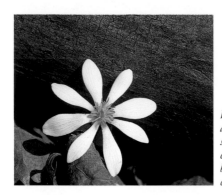

Hot flushes that are associated with severe headaches can be relieved by Sanguinaria canadensis.

SYMPTOMS / MEDICINE

Symptoms	Medicine
❧ Flushing is always followed by sweating.	◉ Amyl nitrosum
❧ The hot flushes are sudden and violent.	◉ Glonoinum
❧ Sudden flushes of heat are followed by nervousness and weakness made worse by the slightest motion.	◉ Digitalis purpurea
❧ Hot flushes are frequent and can precede a headache in which the top of the head feels hot while the feet feel cold.	◉ Lachesis mutus
❧ A feeling of being permanently overheated.	◉ Manganum aceticum
❧ Hot flushes and sweats lead to waking up several times a night. ❧ The sweats continue into the daytime especially in a hot, airless room, so the window is kept open. ❧ The tongue feels dry but there is no thirst.	◉ Pulsatilla

DOSAGE

USE THE 12C POTENCY. TAKE TWICE A DAY UNTIL THE SYMPTOMS HAVE LESSENED FOR APPROXIMATELY 48 HOURS. THE MEDICINE MAY THEN BE STOPPED BUT RESTARTED IF THE SYMPTOMS BEGIN TO RETURN. IF NEW SYMPTOMS DEVELOP, THE MEDICINE MAY NEED TO BE CHANGED.

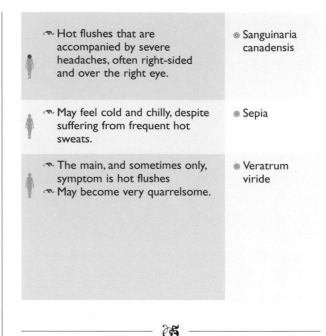

Symptoms	Medicine
❧ Hot flushes that are accompanied by severe headaches, often right-sided and over the right eye.	◉ Sanguinaria canadensis
❧ May feel cold and chilly, despite suffering from frequent hot sweats.	◉ Sepia
❧ The main, and sometimes only, symptom is hot flushes ❧ May become very quarrelsome.	◉ Veratrum viride

❧❦

Prolapse

*W*hen an organ or part of an organ or tissue drops down from its normal position, the condition is called a prolapse. Women most commonly suffer a prolapse of the uterus (womb) which frequently results from straining and stretching the pelvic tissues during childbirth. *This condition requires professional help as surgery may be necessary.*

SYMPTOMS / MEDICINE

Symptoms	Medicine
❧ Prolapse occurs, with a severe bearing-down sensation.	◉ Agaricus muscarius
❧ Prolapse, pain in the left ovary and back. ❧ Heavy periods.	◉ Argentum metallicum

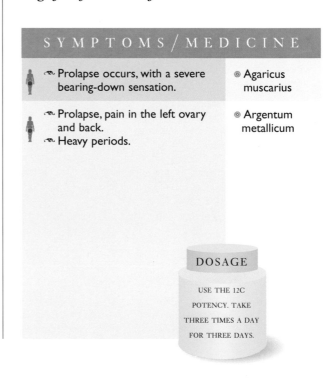

DOSAGE

USE THE 12C POTENCY. TAKE THREE TIMES A DAY FOR THREE DAYS.

Period problems during the menopause

*P*eriods become scanty for some women as they approach the menopause, but you may be unfortunate enough to experience very heavy periods which may also occur at frequent intervals. *Non-menopausal causes of flooding require conventional diagnosis and treatment, and you should consult your doctor about this.* Cancer of the uterus is the most serious cause of flooding or irregular bleeding but it is relatively rare and you are likely to be cured completely if the diagnosis is made early. One of the following medicines may provide help (see also Heavy periods, page 24), but constitutional treatment is sometimes needed.

SYMPTOMS / MEDICINE

Symptoms	Medicine
❧ Marked fatigue and exhaustion.	⊛ Chinchona officinalis
❧ Severe period pain that comes and goes, and is relieved when the period starts. ❧ Frequent hot flushes. ❧ An intolerance of heat, tight clothing and heavy bedclothes. ❧ There have been several previous pregnancies.	⊛ Lachesis mutus
❧ Erratic and scanty periods.	⊛ Manganum aceticum
❧ Heavy periods with dark clots. ❧ The blood flow increases with any movement.	⊛ Medorrhinum
❧ Severe period pain, starting in the lower back and extending to the front. ❧ Loss of gushing, bright red blood. ❧ Symptoms may be relieved by walking about.	⊛ Sabina
❧ Continuous loss of dark, thin blood. ❧ Feels cold but is intolerant of heat.	⊛ Secale cornutum
❧ The periods come early, and are heavy. ❧ A dragging-down feeling as if the contents of the pelvis might fall out. ❧ An aversion to sex or being touched sexually. ❧ Hunger not relieved by eating.	⊛ Sepia
❧ Very heavy periods with dark clots accompanied by dizziness.	⊛ Ustilago maidis

DOSAGE

USE THE 30C POTENCY. TAKE FOUR TIMES A DAY FOR FOUR DAYS WHEN THE BLEEDING STARTS.

Vaginal dryness

*D*ryness of the vagina is a frequent, unpleasant and sometimes distressing condition that often starts during the menopause. It is due to the natural ageing process in the body, which leads to thinning and drying of the vaginal lining. However, it is likely that these symptoms are also related to the hormonal changes of the menopause. It results in painful intercourse, which may place a strain on a woman's relationship with her partner, and an increased susceptibility to vaginal infections. Various lubricating creams, such as KY jelly, are available from most pharmacies and may help to improve the condition in some cases.

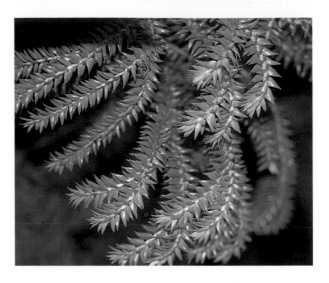

After they have been homeopathically prepared, the spores from Lycopodium clavatum *can heal conditions such as vaginal dryness.*

SYMPTOMS / MEDICINE

Symptoms	Medicine
❧ Vagina is dry, hot and sensitive.	◉ Aconitum napellus
❧ Vagina feels raw and sore. ❧ A vaginal discharge is worse at night. ❧ An involuntary passage of urine with coughing, sneezing and nose-blowing.	◉ Causticum
❧ A dry, hot feeling in vagina. ❧ Vaginal spasm and pain on attempting intercourse.	◉ Ferrum phosphoricum
❧ An extreme vaginal itch. ❧ An acrid, offensive discharge.	◉ Kreosotum
❧ Dryness of vagina leads to soreness during and after intercourse. ❧ An acrid discharge that burns vagina.	◉ Lycopodium clavatum
❧ A dry vagina with an acrid, watery discharge. ❧ Pain after urination and involuntary loss on coughing and walking.	◉ Natrum muriaticum
❧ Intense irritation of vagina and surrounding area, which is made worse by thinking about it. ❧ Breasts and nipples may feel sore and sensitive to touch.	◉ Medorrhinum
❧ Intercourse is painful. ❧ A bearing-down sensation is present and is worse in the evening.	◉ Sepia
❧ Vagina feels dry, hot and itchy.	◉ Tarentula hispana
❧ Erotic sensations may accompany a period. ❧ Intercourse is prevented by the extreme sensitivity of vagina.	◉ Thuja occidentalis

DOSAGE

USE THE 12C POTENCY. TAKE THREE TIMES A DAY UNTIL AN IMPROVEMENT IS MAINTAINED.

Stress incontinence

*A*ccidental leakage of urine often happens when there is sneezing, laughing or coughing. It occurs because the muscle closing the bladder is unable to remain closed. Although it is generally more common in women who have had several children, it is also part of the ageing process.

SYMPTOMS / MEDICINE

Symptoms	Medicine
● Urinary incontinence is worse at night and from coughing. ● The last few drips of urine burn and smart.	◉ Apis mellifica
● Involuntary urination occurs during sleep, when coughing, blowing the nose, or sneezing. ● Problems in starting to urinate and difficulty in passing the last few drops.	◉ Causticum
● Constant incontinence. ● Urine spurts with coughing.	◉ Ferrum phosphoricum
● Involuntary urination occurs when walking or coughing.	◉ Natrum muriaticum
● Tendency to pass a few drops of urine when coughing, when passing wind or after a surprise.	◉ Pulsatilla
● Passes urine when laughing, coughing or sneezing. ● Involuntary urination occurs during first sleep.	◉ Sepia
● Involuntary spurting of urine happens when coughing or sneezing. ● Pain is felt over the bladder.	◉ Zincum metallicum

DOSAGE

USE THE 12C POTENCY. TAKE TWICE A DAY UNTIL AN IMPROVEMENT OCCURS AND IS MAINTAINED.

Osteoporosis

*B*ones, particularly those in the spine and pelvis, lose calcium and become less dense with age. Symptoms vary considerably, and in some women there may be none at all. Usually, however, there is some degree of pain, especially in the back. Thinning of the bones means that fractures occur very easily. When this occurs in the spine, there may be a consequent loss of height. Attention to diet is helpful as an adequate intake of protein, calcium, phosphorus and vitamin D is important. See also page 52–53.

SYMPTOMS / MEDICINE

Symptoms	Medicine
● Rheumatic-type pains are felt after exposure to damp conditions. ● Pain and weakness in the back, especially the lower back. ● Curvature of the upper part of the spine. ● Symptoms improve when lying on the painful area.	◉ Calcarea carbonica
● Stiffness and pain with a cold, numb feeling. ● Pain in the lower back and around the hips, which can be so bad that it may feel as if a bone is broken. ● Pain is worse in changeable weather.	◉ Calcarea phosphorica
● There is weakness in the arms and legs. ● Sciatic pain is felt in the hips, legs and feet. ● Pain is better for warmth and in wet, humid weather.	◉ Silicea
● Useful for treating fractures caused by osteoporosis.	◉ Symphytum officinale

DOSAGE

USE THE 12C POTENCY. TAKE TWICE A DAY FOR FOUR WEEKS, THEN REPEAT WHEN NECESSARY AFTER THIS.

CHAPTER 4

THE HEAD & THROAT

THE HEAD is composed of a bony box (the skull) that contains and protects the brain. The bones at the front of the skull are shaped to provide cavities for the eyes, form the nose and bear the upper teeth. The lower teeth are set in another bone, the jaw, which is hinged from the skull.

HAIR

Each hair on the scalp emerges from its hair follicle, grows by about 1cm/½in each month for about three years, goes into a resting phase that lasts for about three months, drops out and is replaced by a new hair.

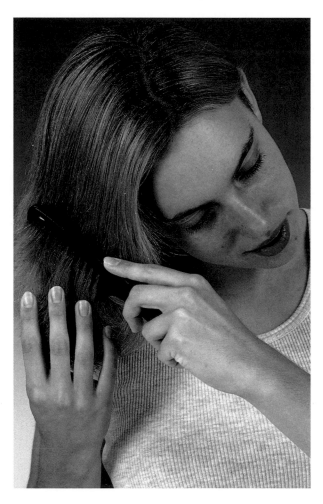

It is normal to shed a 100–150 hairs a day as your hair has its own life cycle of growth and replacement.

On average there are about 300,000 hairs on the scalp, and some 100–150 are shed each day. Dry, brittle hair is usually the result of excessive shampooing, exposure to heat by blow drying or heated rollers, or the application of the chemicals used in perming, bleaching and tinting. Very occasionally dry hair is caused by an underactive thyroid gland or malnutrition. Greasy hair is caused by overactivity of the sebaceous glands (see Skin section, page 98).

EARS

Your ears allow you to hear and are also the organs of balance. The inner ear is connected to the back of the throat by the eustachian tube. Infection spreading through this tube from the throat may cause some loss of hearing, and sometimes affects the balance.

NOSE

In addition to allowing you to detect smells, your nose warms and moistens the air as it is drawn into the lungs. The hairs in the nose trap dust particles and, if necessary, get rid of them by causing you to sneeze and expel them. The most common disorders of the nose are the common cold, flu, sinusitis, hay fever and other types of allergies.

MOUTH

The mouth is the first part of the digestive system. You breathe through your mouth if your nose is blocked or when your body needs more air, for example when running. Your mouth is where the vibrations produced by your vocal cords are converted into speech. Infections in the mouth are common and include mouth ulcers, which often respond well to homeopathy. Cysts can occur in the mouth when the small glands that produce mucus become blocked: these usually clear by themselves. However, any lump or sore that persists for more than one month should always be checked by your doctor or dentist.

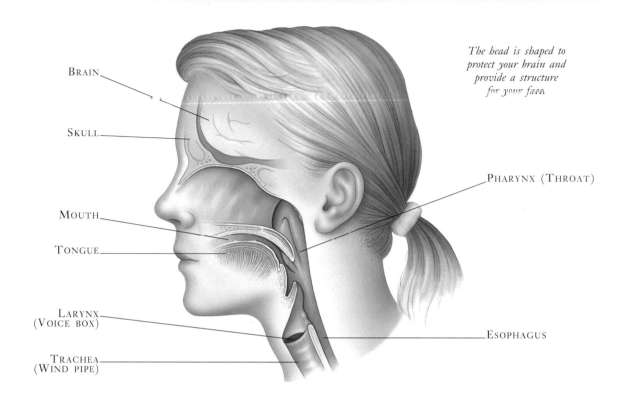

The head is shaped to protect your brain and provide a structure for your face.

BRAIN

SKULL

PHARYNX (THROAT)

MOUTH

TONGUE

LARYNX
(VOICE BOX)

ESOPHAGUS

TRACHEA
(WIND PIPE)

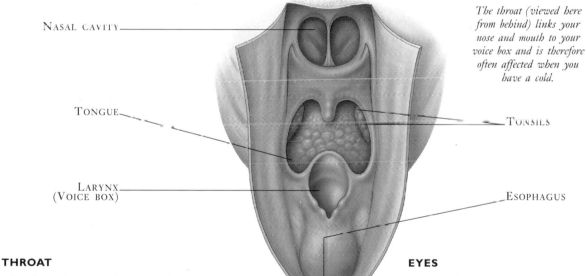

The throat (viewed here from behind) links your nose and mouth to your voice box and is therefore often affected when you have a cold.

NASAL CAVITY

TONGUE

TONSILS

LARYNX
(VOICE BOX)

ESOPHAGUS

THROAT

The throat is a popular name for the pharynx. This is the area that connects your nose and mouth to the larynx (voice box) and esophagus. The pharynx contains the adenoids which, together with the tonsils at the back of the mouth, help to fight back against infection. A sore throat is a very common symptom that is caused by inflammation in the pharynx or tonsils, usually as the result of an infection. It may be the first symptom that is noticed with the common cold, flu or with glandular fever (infectious mononucleosis).

EYES

The eyes are the organs of sight and they work in unison to provide you with two slightly different views of an object. These are interpreted by the brain to give a sense of depth that enables you to judge distances. Homeopathic treatment can be very helpful when the eyes become red and inflamed from infection (conjunctivitis) or as a result of an allergy. However, it is best to check the diagnosis first with your doctor. Urgent medical assessment is vital for painful red eyes, especially when they occur in older people.

A QUICK GUIDE TO TREATING COLDS AND INFLUENZA

Colds and flu respond best when tackled early. This guide will help you to use the homeopathic medicines you are likely to have in the home already.

TO USE THE GUIDE

1 Choose which heading(s) (A–G) most closely describe(s) your illness.

2 Select a medicine using this and the *Materia Medica* section of this book (pages 145–171).

3 Take the medicine, at 6c or 30c potency, two hourly for up to six doses.

4 Decrease frequency as symptoms improve.

5 Try another medicine if the symptoms persist or alter.

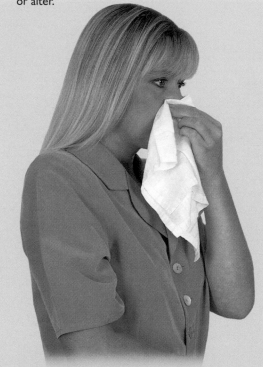

To help relieve the symptoms, homeopathic medicine should be started at the very first sign of a cold or flu.

A. SUDDEN ONSET WITH HIGH FEVER
ACONITUM NAPELLUS

☙ After exposure to a cold wind or due to shock.

☙ Restlessness, anxiety and a great need for being in the fresh air.

☙ A runny nose.

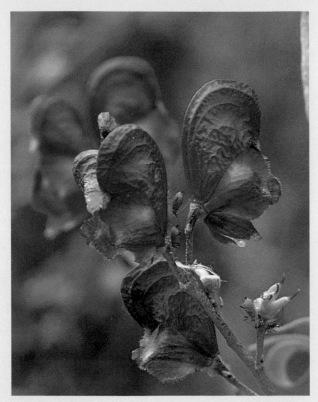

Aconitum napellus is often the best medicine for an infection that comes on very suddenly after being out in a cold wind.

BELLADONNA

☙ A very red face with dilated pupils.

☙ When every movement is painful.

☙ When darkness, quiet and warmth are sought.

☙ When there is headache and a blocked nose.

Aconitum napellus and Belladonna tend to work best in the first 48 hours; after this a change of medicine is advisable.

B. MORE GRADUAL ONSET AND LESS FEVER
FERRUM PHOSPHORICUM

☙ May be flushed but want cold compresses.

☙ There may be a nosebleed.

C. INFECTION STARTS WITH SNEEZING AND COPIOUS CLEAR OR WHITISH DISCHARGE
NATRUM MURIATICUM

☙ Hatred of fuss, love of salt and may weep alone.

☙ If the condition is worse in cold air.

☙ Often there is an attack of cold sores.

D. STARTS WITH CREEPING CHILLINESS

MERCURIUS SOLUBILIS

- ❧ Sneezing with a burning, green discharge.
- ❧ Symptoms are worse in a warm room but hatred of the cold.
- ❧ Profuse sweats occuring that do not improve any of the symptoms.
- ❧ Great thirst despite copious saliva.

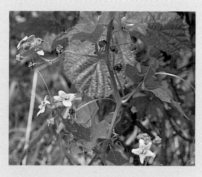

The large, white and poisonous root of Bryonia alba is used to make this useful homeopathic medicine which can help relieve flu or colds that start in the nose.

E. STARTS IN THE NOSE AND
MOVES RAPIDLY TO THE THROAT AND CHEST

BRYONIA

- ❧ Irritability and a desire to be at home, lie still and be left alone.
- ❧ Very thirsty and a craving for long drinks.
- ❧ A dry, painful cough

F. SHIVERY AND UNABLE TO GET WARM

ARSENICUM ALBUM

- ❧ Restless, anxious and fussy feelings.
- ❧ Unable to get warm, but likes head to be in the fresh air.
- ❧ There is a thin, watery discharge from the nose, which burns the nose and upper lip.
- ❧ Nose remains blocked despite discharge.

GELSEMIUM SEMPERVIRENS

- ❧ Tiredness in both mind and body, with chills up and down the spine.
- ❧ Slow onset of symptoms, in mild, damp weather.
- ❧ Lack of thirst.

NUX VOMICA

- ❧ Feelings of oversensitivity, irritability, touchiness and sensitivity to any draft.
- ❧ For sudden infection caused by cold, dry weather.
- ❧ Nose is blocked at night, and there is discharge by day or in a warm room.

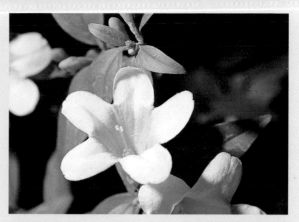

Gelsemium sempervirens, to be taken with shivery cold or flu symptoms, is derived from the beautiful plant.

G. A DESIRE FOR OPEN AIR

ALLIUM CEPA

- ❧ Streaming eyes (bland tears) as well as nose (burning discharge).
- ❧ Hot and thirsty.

PULSATILLA

- ❧ Weepy and wants sympathy, but feels better for gentle exercise.
- ❧ Thirstless
- ❧ Catarrh is greenish and contains pus.
- ❧ Nose is blocked at night and indoors.

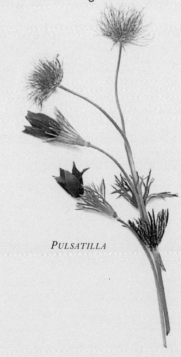

PULSATILLA

Headaches and migraine

Headaches can develop for many different reasons. The main causes of repeated headaches are stress and tension, the beginning of a period, eyestrain, sinusitis and raised blood pressure. In many people headaches occur for no apparent reason. Migraines usually need constitutional treatment but one of the following medicines may be helpful. *If a severe headache occurs frequently or fails to resolve easily, a doctor should always be consulted.*

DOSAGE

USE THE 12C POTENCY. TAKE FOUR TIMES A DAY WHEN NECESSARY.

SYMPTOMS / MEDICINE	
Frequent headaches and palpitations.	⊛ Amyl nitrosum
A headache which feels as if there is a weight on the top of the head.	⊛ Cactus grandiflorus
Frequent throbbing or shooting headaches.	⊛ Cimicifuga racemosa
A throbbing, pulsating headache that is worse for the first two days of a period.	⊛ Crocus sativus
A throbbing headache that is worsened or caused by being in the sun. Frequent dizzy attacks are experienced.	⊛ Glonoinum
Hot flushes are frequent and can precede a headache in which the top of the head feels hot while the feet feel cold. Skin appears blue/purple, especially during a hot flush.	⊛ Lachesis mutus
Frequent hot flushes accompanied by severe headaches, often right-sided, over the eye.	⊛ Sanguinaria canadensis
For persistent headaches after a head injury.	⊛ Natrum sulphuricum

Cold sores

Cold sores are small, fluid-filled blisters that develop around the mouth. They are due to infection by the *Herpes simplex* virus and can be difficult to get rid of completely as the virus remains dormant in the skin. Common causes of cold sores are dental treatment, sunlight and physical or emotional stress.

SYMPTOMS / MEDICINE	
Extreme thirst. Mouth may be sore and inflamed.	⊛ Capsicum annuum
Tongue is dry and the surface feels rough. A sore throat with thick, sticky saliva, which tastes soapy. Symptoms are worsened by the cold	⊛ Dulcamara
Mouth feels dry, while the tongue and lips are numb and dry and may tingle. A crack in the middle of the lower lip.	⊛ Natrum muriaticum
Blisters around the mouth, which may extend to the chin. The corners of the mouth ulcerate. Tongue has a red tip, feels sore and may be coated and cracked.	⊛ Rhus toxicodendron

DOSAGE

USE THE 12C POTENCY. TAKE FOUR TIMES A DAY FOR FOUR DAYS.

Bad breath

Halitosis

When it has been present for some time without clearing spontaneously, bad breath is usually caused by bad teeth or catarrhal conditions of the nose, throat or sinuses. It may also indicate some kind of disorder of the gastro-intestinal tract, such as mouth ulcers or an upset in the stomach. People who breathe through the mouth or who are smokers often tend to suffer from halitosis. The breath may also smell unpleasant for a while after eating highly flavored or highly spiced food.

SYMPTOMS/MEDICINE

- A bitter or putrid taste in the mouth.
- Girls at puberty are particularly affected.
- Ulcers may develop on the gums.

⊛ Aurum metallicum

- Tongue feels burnt and is dry and brown with red shiny edge.
- Food tastes flat and bitter
- Breath is foul.
- Only liquids can be swallowed.

⊛ Baptisia tinctoria

- Breath smells mouldy.
- Mouth and tongue ulcers hurt when eating salty or sour foods.
- Mouth feels hot, dry and tender.

⊛ Borax

DOSAGE

USE THE 6C POTENCY. TAKE FOUR TIMES A DAY UNTIL AN IMPROVEMENT OCCURS, THEN STOP. REPEAT AS AND WHEN NECESSARY.

- Thick, offensive, dry, green-yellow crusts form on the back of the mouth.
- Swallowing is difficult.
- Breath is foul.

⊛ Elaps corallinus

- Breath smells like urine.
- Sour-tasting belches.
- Burning blisters are found on the tongue.

⊛ Graphites

- Excessive salivation and saliva tastes metallic – like copper.
- Gums become spongy, sore and bleed easily.
- Tongue is yellow, flabby and thick.
- Teeth indentations form on the sides of the tongue.
- Breath has an offensive smell.

⊛ Mercurius solubilis

- A dry mouth with no thirst that is worse in the morning.
- Tongue is yellow or white and covered by a tenacious mucus.
- Breath is offensive.

⊛ Pulsatilla

- Bad breath comes from infected gums.

⊛ Silicea

- Breath is offensive and smells of onions.
- Hot, sour-tasting belches.
- Tongue is fissured and painful.
- A foul odour from the mouth from excessive mucus at the back of the throat.

⊛ Sinapis nigra

- An offensive taste in the mouth.

⊛ Spigelia anthelmia

- Tongue is dry, red, sore and shiny, with a burning sensation at its tip.
- Breath feels cold and smells foul.

⊛ Terebinthina

- Chronic nasal catarrh produces bad breath and a mouldy taste.
- A loss of the sense of smell.

⊛ Teucrium marum

Hoarseness

Laryngitis

Acute inflammation of the larynx (voice box) from infection interferes with its normal function and produces hoarseness or even a complete loss of voice. Overuse of the voice by singing, public speaking or something similar can lead to the same symptoms being experienced. ***If laryngitis does not respond to treatment, or lasts for more than 14 days, always consult a doctor for advice.***

SYMPTOMS / MEDICINE

Symptoms	Medicine
• Temperature is raised, throat feels rough and voice becomes hoarse. • Thin, frothy sputum.	◉ Aconitum napellus
• Burning rawness in the throat and there is total voice loss.	◉ Ammonium causticum
• Rawness and burning in the larynx. • Copious mucus which looks like boiled starch is produced, but is easily coughed up. • For chronic laryngitis that is common in singers.	◉ Argentum metallicum
• Voice suddenly changes. • A painful, dry cough with hoarseness and rawness from overuse of the voice.	◉ Arum triphyllum
• Hoarseness is sudden, with a red, dry throat and an aversion to drinking.	◉ Belladonna
• Worse in the evening and after exposure to damp.	◉ Carbo vegetabilis
• Complete voice loss with dryness in the larynx. • Worse in the morning. • Rawness is felt under the breastbone. • A dry, hollow cough that is relieved by a cold drink.	◉ Causticum
• Slight fever. • A slight cough. • A small amount of mucus is coughed up. • All symptoms are worse in a draft.	◉ Hepar sulphuris calcareum
• Worse in the evening, larynx hurts when talking and voice sounds rough and hoarse.	◉ Phosphorus
• Throat feels very dry and talking is painful. • Chest also feels sore and there is an unproductive cough.	◉ Senega officinalis
• Harsh barking cough. • Throat is sensitive to touch and is worse when in bed.	◉ Spongia tosta

CAUSTICUM

Mouth ulcers

*M*outh ulcers can occur as a result of infection, either in the mouth or elsewhere in the body, as a result of such conditions as throat infections, thrush, measles, glandular fever and the *Herpes* *simplex* virus, which produces cold sores. They may also develop from a shortage of vitamins B or C, with some anaemias, mechanical trauma from ill-fitting dentures or jagged teeth, and excess alcohol, tobacco and hot, spicy foods. Some types of drugs can also cause mouth ulcers, as can individual sensitivities to different tooth-pastes or mouthwashes.

SYMPTOMS / MEDICINE

Symptoms	Medicine
❧ Ulcers on the roof of the mouth.	◉ Agaricus muscarius
❧ Ulceration in the mouth with dryness and a burning sensation. ❧ Gums are unhealthy and bleed easily.	◉ Arsenicum album
❧ Mouth feels hot and tender, the ulcers bleed on touch and when eating.	◉ Borax
❧ Small white ulcers develop in the mouth and throat. ❧ Burning sensation in the mouth, pharynx and throat, with difficulty in swallowing liquids.	◉ Cantharis
❧ Tongue becomes covered in small white ulcers.	◉ Carbo vegetabilis
❧ Gums and mouth are painful, and gums bleed easily when touched. ❧ Ulcers form in the corners of the mouth.	◉ Hepar sulphuris calcareum
❧ Ulcers are white, tongue is coated grey-white and neck glands become enlarged.	◉ Kali muriaticum
❧ White, raw, burning ulcers, causing foul breath. ❧ Gums become swollen, spongy and bleed. ❧ Tongue is dry and cracked at the tip and catches on the teeth.	◉ Lachesis mutus
❧ Ulcers occur in the mouth and throat, salivation is increased and the gums become spongy and recede.	◉ Mercurius solubilis
❧ Small white ulcers develop in mouth and gums appear white and swollen and bleed easily, producing blood in the saliva.	◉ Nux vomica
❧ Gums are sore, tongue is red and cracked and ulcers form at the corners of the mouth. ❧ Blisters develop around the mouth and chin.	◉ Rhus toxicodendron
❧ Ulceration in mouth and at the back of throat, with a dry, burning sensation. ❧ Tongue is white and feels scalded.	◉ Sanguinaria canadensis
❧ Tongue is white with small white ulcers on it and in mouth. ❧ Saliva has a metallic taste and breath is foul.	◉ Sarsaparilla

DOSAGE

USE THE 30C POTENCY. TAKE FOUR TIMES A DAY UNTIL AN IMPROVEMENT OCCURS, THEN STOP. REPEAT AS AND WHEN NECESSARY

Sore throat and tonsillitis

*A*lthough many healthy throats are red (more so in smokers), a sore, red throat with a raised temperature is indicative of infection and may precede acute tonsillitis. Other illnesses in which there may be a sore, red throat are influenza, the common cold, glandular fever (infectious mononucleosis) and adenoid infections. The tonsils, which are on both sides of the back of the mouth, can become acutely inflamed, often quite suddenly. Symptoms of tonsillitis include a sore throat and fever, and all cases have a discharge of pus on the tonsils. Offensive breath and a coated tongue are also usually present. *If there is no response to homeopathic medicine within 24 to 36 hours, consult a doctor immediately.*

SYMPTOMS / MEDICINE

Symptoms	Medicine
◦ A sensation as if a splinter is stuck in the throat when swallowing. ◦ Throat is dark red, rough and sore.	⊛ Argentum nitricum
◦ Tonsils are both inflamed and sore. ◦ Smarting pain occurs when swallowing. ◦ Colds always develop into tonsillitis. ◦ Neck glands and glands behind ears are enlarged. ◦ Chronic tonsil enlargement occurs.	⊛ Baryta carbonica
◦ The condition comes and goes suddenly. ◦ Hot red skin and also a dry mouth. ◦ Constant desire to swallow but no desire to drink. ◦ Throat is bright red with much pus and exudate on the tonsils, especially the right. ◦ Swallowing is difficult and produces sharp pains which are felt in the tonsils.	⊛ Belladonna
◦ Throat is very inflamed and with a feeling of constriction. ◦ Throat feels as if it is on fire.	⊛ Cantharis
◦ Pain which extends to ears. ◦ A smoker's sore throat with a burning, smarting sensation. ◦ Cold aggravates condition.	⊛ Capsicum annuum
◦ A rough, scraping sensation in the throat develops after catching cold in damp weather.	⊛ Dulcamara
◦ Useful if taken early in the attack. ◦ A violent burning headache with aching limbs. ◦ Throat feels hot.	⊛ Guaiacum
◦ A sensation of having a splinter in the throat, which feels raw, as if scraped. ◦ Tonsils are both inflamed and swollen. ◦ Useful for shaking and chills. ◦ Pus on the tonsils.	⊛ Hepar sulphuris calcareum
◦ There is tearing pain with a chronic sore throat. ◦ Mucus sticks in the throat. ◦ Tonsils are dark red or purple in colour. ◦ A lot of external swelling and tenderness. ◦ It starts on the left side. ◦ Pain shoots to the ear when swallowing. ◦ Hot drinks cause aggravation.	⊛ Lachesis mutus
◦ Rarely needed at the onset, use when pus is present with thick, tenacious saliva and foul breath. ◦ Tonsils are very swollen and dark red in colour.	⊛ Mercurius solubilis
◦ White patches on throat with sharp, sore, stinging pain making swallowing difficult.	⊛ Nitricum acidum
◦ Pain is worse when coughing. ◦ An ulcerated sore throat.	⊛ Phosphorus
◦ Throat feels hot, and pain at the tongue's root goes to the ear. ◦ Tonsils are large and dark blue/purple. ◦ Intense dryness, smarting and burning in the throat.	⊛ Phytolacca decandra

DOSAGE

USE THE 30C POTENCY. TAKE FOUR TIMES A DAY FOR THREE DAYS.

Cataracts

Cataract is the term used to describe the clouding of the lens of the eye. It is like looking through frosted glass; you can still see light, but you cannot see objects clearly. It is most common in older people but it can be present from birth or follow an injury. Recent research has shown that you can decrease the risk of developing cataracts by eating foods which are rich in beta-carotene (red and green vegetables and fruits, particularly spinach, sweet potatoes and winter squash) and vitamin E (including broccoli, almonds and wheatgerm). *Consult a doctor.*

DOSAGE

USE THE 6C POTENCY. TAKE TWICE A DAY FOR A MONTH. IF THE VISION SEEMS BETTER, STOP FOR A WEEK AND REPEAT THE COURSE.

SYMPTOMS / MEDICINE

Symptoms	Medicine
ᴑ Feeling that there is a net curtain before the eyes. ᴑ Objects seem far off.	◉ Carbo animalis
ᴑ A dimness of vision while reading. ᴑ A dimness of vision as if looking through a mist.	◉ Calcarea carbonica
ᴑ There is a sensation of a veil covering everything. ᴑ Vision is improved by shading eyes with the hand.	◉ Phosphorus

CALCAREA CARBONICA

Toothache

Toothache is often the result of dental caries (decay) which, if deep enough, can cause inflammation of the pulp of the tooth or even a dental abscess. Inflammation and infection in the gums cause pain and can result in the tooth becoming extremely sensitive to temperature change, or sweet food, as the gum recedes and the root of the tooth becomes exposed. *You should see your dental surgeon for diagnosis and treatment.*

SYMPTOMS / MEDICINE

Symptoms	Medicine
ᴑ Pain is caused by exposure to cold wind.	◉ Aconitum napellus
ᴑ Toothache following dental treatment, or injury.	◉ Arnica montana
ᴑ Frantic pain, made worse by anger. ᴑ Pain is aggravated by coffee and warm drinks.	◉ Chamomilla
ᴑ Toothache is relieved by ice cold water.	◉ Coffea cruda
ᴑ Very sensitive to the pain and also to any cold air or draft.	◉ Hepar sulphuris calcareum
ᴑ Toothache occurs during pregnancy. ᴑ Pain is worse at night and from the cold.	◉ Magnesia carbonica
ᴑ Toothache is relieved by heat and warm drinks. ᴑ Pain is much worse after going to bed.	◉ Magnesia phosphorica
ᴑ Gingivitis and toothache are associated with excessive production of saliva.	◉ Mercurius solubilis
ᴑ Pain is made much worse by warmth.	◉ Pulsatilla
ᴑ Pain is aggravated by cold and by eating. ᴑ Pain is worse during a period.	◉ Staphysagria

DOSAGE

USE THE 30C POTENCY. REPEAT EVERY TWO HOURS UNTIL RELIEF OCCURS.

Redness of the eyes and eyelids

*C*onjunctivitis is the inflammation of the outer covering of the eye (conjunctiva) as a result of allergy or infection. The symptoms are redness, discomfort and discharge in the eyes. If you are not better 24 hours after using a homeopathic medicine, you should see your doctor. *Conditions that cause the eye(s) to be painful and red are sometimes serious, so you should always consult your doctor urgently.*

SYMPTOMS / MEDICINE

Symptoms	Medicine
➤ Stinging, burning discomfort in the eyes that is relieved by cold compresses. ➤ Swollen pinkish lids.	⊛ Apis mellifica
➤ Copious and frequent discharge of pus. ➤ Conjunctiva is swollen and scarlet.	⊛ Argentum nitricum
➤ There is a burning, watery discharge, relieved by warm application.	⊛ Arsenicum album
➤ A marked intolerance of light. ➤ Little discharge.	⊛ Euphrasia officinalis
➤ A bland profuse discharge that is white or yellow. ➤ Condition is better in the open air, but worse in a warm room.	⊛ Pulsatilla

DOSAGE

USE THE 6C POTENCY. TAKE HOURLY FOR UP TO 12 HOURS.

Blepharitis

*B*lepharitis is a condition in which the eyelids are inflamed, red and often itchy and scaling. It is sometimes associated with eczema or dandruff and the eyes can also be reddish. You should try to remove the scales with cotton moistened with warm water and then apply some Calendula cream.

SYMPTOMS / MEDICINE

Symptoms	Medicine
➤ Eyelids are gummy, crusty and sticky. ➤ A desire to rub the eyelids.	⊛ Borax
➤ Red and swollen eyelids that are sticky in the morning.	⊛ Graphites
➤ Eyelids are red and are sensitive to both the wind and cold air.	⊛ Hepar sulphuris calcareum
➤ Eyelids are both inflamed and sticky. ➤ Condition is aggravated by windy weather.	⊛ Pulsatilla
➤ Eyelids feel sticky and the discharge is acidic. ➤ Edges of the eyelids are red in color.	⊛ Psorinum
➤ Eyes are sensitive to light. ➤ A feeling of dryness under the eyelids.	⊛ Sanicula
➤ Edges of the eyelids are dry and scaly. ➤ Eyelids stick together at night.	⊛ Thuja occidentalis

DOSAGE

USE THE 6C POTENCY. TAKE FOUR TIMES A DAY FOR UP TO THREE WEEKS.

Styes

Styes are small boils that occur in the eyelid. Irritation of the eyelid affected is often the first sign that is noticed, and it is soon followed by redness, pain and swelling.

SYMPTOMS	MEDICINE
For recurrent styes. Eyelid becomes swollen, and sharp, piercing pains develop. Conjunctiva becomes red.	Apis mellifica
Eyelids are dry, red and scaly and there is intolerance of artificial light.	Graphites
For styes in the inner corner of the eye (nearest the nose). Eyelids become red and ulcerate.	Lycopodium clavatum
A thick, profuse, yellow discharge. Eyelids become inflamed and stick together. Eyes itch and burn.	Pulsatilla
Eye feels tender to the touch. There is an aversion to the light as it causes sharp pains which run through the eye.	Silicea
Margins of the eye itch. Eyes appear sunken. For recurrent styes.	Staphysagria
Eyelids stick overnight and are dry and scaly.	Thuja occidentalis

Dandruff

Dandruff is the shedding of flakes of dead skin from the scalp. These may be seen in the hair or on the clothes. The condition is harmless but may be aggravated by failure to rinse away products, such as setting lotion or mousse, completely. Occasionally, there is also an itchy, scaly rash, seborrhoeic dermatitis, that can spread to the face and upper body.

SYMPTOMS	MEDICINE
Scalp is rough and dry. Scalp is very itchy, especially at night.	Arsenicum album
There are large scales of dead skin. Hair loss is noticed when combing the hair.	Cantharis
There are yellowish scales of dead skin. A moist sticky rash.	Kali suphuricum
White scales and crusting at the hair margins. Greasy hair.	Natrum muriaticum
Itchy dandruff combined with dry skin. May be some hair loss.	Phosphorus
Scalp is dry and sore or burning after being scratched. Dandruff is worse in the heat and at night.	Sulphur
White, scaly dandruff. Hair is very dry.	Thuja occidentalis

Hair loss

The most common form of baldness is the slow but progressive loss of hair that affects men and, occasionally, older women. It involves the gradual loss of hair and usually starts on the crown and at the temples. Another form of hair loss called *Alopecia areata* may develop in older children and adults. In this condition small bald patches develop fairly quickly over a few days or weeks and may slowly enlarge. After about 6 to 10 weeks, fine hair starts to grow again and within about two months has returned to normal. Sudden loss of hair may also be caused by extreme mental stress or trauma, but this is very rare.

SYMPTOMS / MEDICINE	
✎ Scalp itches and feels numb.	◉ Alumina
✎ Hair loss occurring in the very young or very old, especially in shy people who have little self-confidence.	◉ Baryta carbonica
✎ Premature baldness with greying of the hair occuring at an early age.	◉ Lycopodium clavatum
✎ Oily sweating of the scalp with associated loss of hair.	◉ Mercurius solubilis
✎ Baldness following acute, debilitating illnesses.	◉ Thallium metallicum
✎ Moist eczema appears on the head and face with extreme itching and the appearance of bald spots.	◉ Vinca minor

DOSAGE

USE THE 6C POTENCY. TAKE TWICE A DAY UNTIL AN IMPROVEMENT OCCURS.

Hay fever

This sometimes distressing condition is caused by an allergy to one or more pollens and mostly occurs in the spring and summer. The main symptoms, which are due to an irritation of the nose and eye membranes, are bouts of violent sneezing with watery eyes. The nose may also run, but this may alternate with a stuffed-up nose. Other symptoms that may develop are itching of the roof of the mouth, itching in the ears and, in some patients, a mild form of asthma with a sensation of tightness in the chest.

If the cause of the allergy is known, it is useful to take a potency of it during the winter months to desensitize the sufferer. The more common causes of hay fever are all available for this purpose and may be obtained from homeopathic pharmacies. In most cases Mixed pollens 30c is the remedy required. For desensitization take the selected desensitizer three times a day on the same day each week four months before the start of the hay fever season (from December) until the season starts.

SYMPTOMS / MEDICINE	
✎ Eyes may swell and sting, although the tears are bland. ✎ Nasal discharge is acrid so that the nose and upper lip become sore. ✎ Frequent sneezing. ✎ Headache at the back of the head often accompanies the hay fever. ✎ Worse indoors and in the evening.	◉ Allium cepa
✎ Eyes feel burning hot and the tears are acrid and sting the cheeks. ✎ A thin burning nasal discharge, which burns the top lip. ✎ Nose frequently feels blocked. ✎ A tickling sensation develops in one spot in the nose and is not helped by the violent sneezing which may occur. ✎ Feels worn out and is much better indoors and for warmth.	◉ Arsenicum album

- Pain develops over root of the nose.
- Frequent sneezing with a burning nasal discharge, and nose also feels stuffed up.
- Sneezing is worse at night.

⊛ Arum triphyllum

- Itching in the eyes, nose and roof of the mouth.
- A thin, watery nasal discharge, which later becomes thicker and yellow-green in color.

⊛ Arundo mauritanica

- Condition comes on late in the summer or even in the autumn.
- Eyes swell and produce tears.
- Constant sneezing, and although nose runs, it feels blocked.
- Skin feels hot and dry.
- Better at rest and indoors, much worse after rain.

⊛ Dulcamara

- Eyes burn, itch and run with burning tears.
- Profuse, watery, but bland nasal discharge.
- Frequent sneezing is worse in the evening and at night, but a cough, which may develop, is worse during the day and often goes away at night.

⊛ Euphrasia officinalis

- Eyes feel hot and heavy and look bloodshot.
- Nose runs and produces a burning discharge, mainly in the morning.
- Nose tingles and there is violent sneezing.
- Throat feels dry and burning, face feels hot and the limbs ache.
- Swallowing produces pain in ears.
- Excessive sweats and all the symptoms are worse in the morning.

⊛ Gelsemium sempervirens

- Eyes smart and swell with burning, profuse tears.
- Pain in the sinuses as well as the hay fever.
- Profuse nasal discharge, at first thin, watery and burning, becomes thick, yellow and offensive.
- Violent sneezing.
- Nose becomes red, tender and sore.
- Feels alternately hot and chilly, and worse in the mornings and evenings.

⊛ Kali iodatum

- Eyelids become swollen and itchy.
- Profuse tears that sting the eyes.
- Frequent violent sneezing accompanies a burning, profuse, watery nasal discharge.
- Symptoms are much worse around 10 am.

⊛ Natrum muriaticum

- Eyes and nose itch terribly and the irritation goes to the throat.
- Frequent sneezing in distressing prolonged bouts.
- A watery nasal discharge is much worse indoors, but nose becomes blocked when outdoors and at night.
- Face feels very hot, but can also feel chilly and become bad-tempered.

⊛ Nux vomica

- Eyelids feel hot and become red, although the excess tears are bland.
- Nasal discharge is thin at first, but becomes thicker and then the nose feels sore and blocked.
- Prolonged attacks of violent sneezing which may cause a severe headache and nosebleeds.
- Symptoms are made worse by the odor of apples, garlic, onions and flowers.

⊛ Sabadilla

- A dry throat, which itches and feels swollen.
- Swallowing is difficult.
- A constant desire to swallow saliva.

⊛ Wyethia helenioides

DOSAGE

USE THE 12C POTENCY. TAKE EVERY HALF HOUR UNTIL AN IMPROVEMENT OCCURS, THEN STOP UNTIL THE SYMPTOMS REAPPEAR, AND TAKE AGAIN IN THE SAME WAY.

CHAPTER 5

THE CHEST, HEART & CIRCULATION

THE CHEST

The protective outside wall of the chest is sometimes called the rib cage and the floor of this cage is formed by the diaphragm, which is the sheet of muscle that separates the chest from the abdomen. The ribs are attached to the spine at the back and to the breastbone, or sternum, in front. Breathing is controlled by the diaphragm and by the muscles of the chest wall. As the diaphragm moves down and the ribs are pulled outwards, air is drawn into the lungs through the windpipe (trachea), which divides into two bronchi, one for each lung, inside the chest.

THE LUNGS

The lungs are sponge-like organs that lie on either side of the heart. The air entering the lungs is drawn into smaller and smaller passages as the bronchi divide and branch into bronchioles, which eventually end in thin-walled sacs, the alveoli. The alveoli are surrounded by a network of small blood vessels that absorb oxygen from the air in exchange for carbon dioxide, which is a waste product. Infection is probably still the most common cause of disease in the chest, but asthma is occurring with increasing frequency for reasons that are not clearly understood, although environmental pollution may be a factor. Lung cancer and emphysema are also becoming increasingly common in women.

The risk of heart disease can be reduced by regular exercise: it is never too late to start.

THE HEART

The heart is about the size of a clenched fist and lies at the front of the chest behind the breast bone. It is the muscular pump at the center of the circulatory or cardiovascular system, and it pumps the blood around your body through the arteries and veins. Heart disease is one of the most common causes of death, particularly in older people. It is rare before the menopause, but this is the time when you can do most to prevent it, or at least postpone its onset. If you smoke, the single most important step is to stop. Your heart will be much healthier if you eat a good diet and take regular exercise. Recent research has shown that even if your heart is damaged, it can repair itself better than doctors once thought, so it is never too late to start a healthy lifestyle.

THE BLOOD

The blood distributes oxygen and the products of digestion to where they are needed and also transports waste products to where they can be

THE HEART AND LUNGS

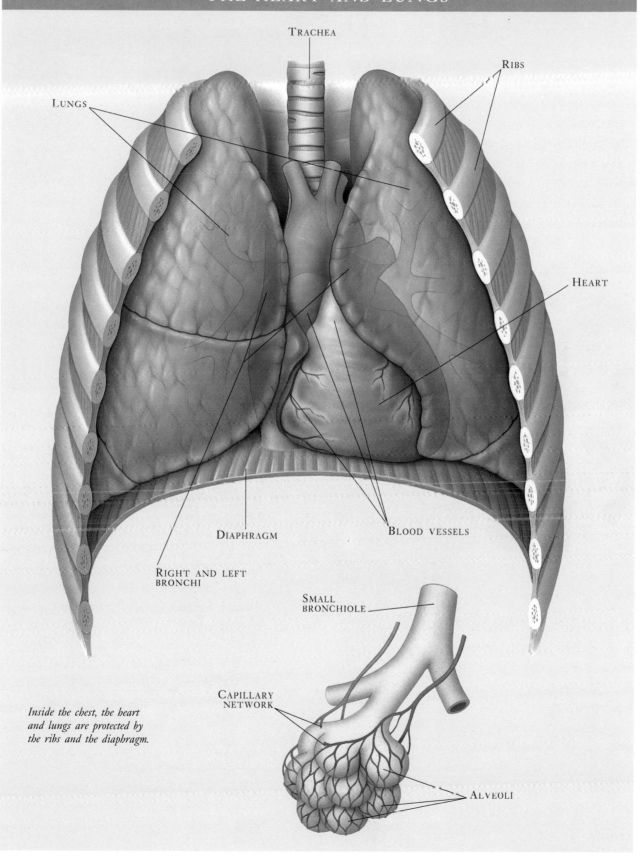

TRACHEA

RIBS

LUNGS

HEART

DIAPHRAGM

BLOOD VESSELS

RIGHT AND LEFT BRONCHI

SMALL BRONCHIOLE

CAPILLARY NETWORK

ALVEOLI

Inside the chest, the heart and lungs are protected by the ribs and the diaphragm.

discharged from the body. It brings white cells and antibodies to fight infection wherever it occurs. Anemia is the most common blood disorder to affect women. Before the menopause, blood is lost in the monthly period and during childbirth. Iron and vitamins needed to make blood are also lost to the baby in pregnancy. Although pallor can be a sign of anemia, it is not always present, and anemic women may simply find they are unusually tired, short of breath or experiencing palpitations. If you think you may be anemic, you should consult your doctor; there are several types of anaemia and it is important to diagnose the cause.

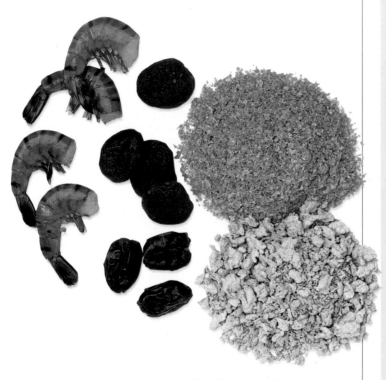

Anemia is the most common blood disorder to affect women. So, plenty of foods that are rich in iron such as shrimp, dried fruit, bran and soy products should be included in the daily diet.

BLOOD VESSELS

The tendency to varicose veins and hemorrhoids is to some extent inherited, but most women suffer some problems with these during pregnancy, when the growing baby puts pressure on the large veins taking blood back to the heart. This causes the walls of the smaller veins to become distended, producing hemorrhoids in the rectum and varicose veins in the legs.

GIVING UP SMOKING

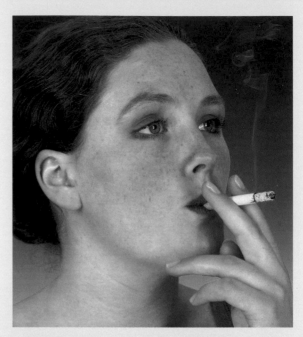

Smokers may reduce their fertility levels and have smaller babies who suffer from learning difficulties later in life.

Every five minutes someone in the U.S.A dies from a disease caused by smoking. Almost all these people die prematurely, and some are babies whose mothers smoked. Non-smokers generally live longer, healthier lives.

DISEASES RELATED TO SMOKING

- Heart attacks: particularly if you have also taken oral contraceptives for a long time.
- Circulatory disorders: aneurysms, strokes (especially those who have used birth control pills), gangrene.
- Cancers: lung, mouth, nose, throat, larynx, esphagus, stomach, liver, pancreas, kidney, bladder, cervix and blood (leukemia).
- Chest diseases: chronic bronchitis, emphysema, recurrent infections.
- Ulcers of stomach and duodenum: more common and take longer to heal.
- Defective vision (tobacco amblyopia).

OTHER RISKS

WOMEN SMOKERS ARE MORE AT RISK OF:

- Reduced fertility: conception takes longer, the risk of ectopic (tubal) pregnancy risk is doubled.

- Complications of pregnancy: miscarriage, premature labor and hemorrhage.
- Period problems: they can be irregular, prolonged, heavy and also painful.
- Early menopause: increased risk of osteoporosis and heart disease (see pages 52–53 and page 74).
- Having low birth-weight babies who may later have learning difficulties.

PASSIVE SMOKING

(LIVING IN A SMOKY ENVIRONMENT)

- Health problems occur particularly in young children. These include respiratory infections such as pneumonia, asthma and allergies.
- Babies are more likely to suffer crib death.

PLANNING A CAMPAIGN
TO QUIT SMOKING

WRITE DOWN THE FOLLOWING LISTS AND KEEP THEM SOMEWHERE HANDY.

- Your reasons for quitting smoking.
- Plans to change your routine for the times that you normally smoke.
- Plans to avoid weight gain (if this could be a problem for you) by . . .
a) Increasing the exercise you take.
b) Avoiding eating when you would normally smoke.
- Plans to use the money you save for rewards, e.g. after a day, a week, a month and six months. Avoid food rewards; clothes or vacations are better.

THINK ABOUT WHAT
HELP YOU MIGHT NEED

- Something for your mouth, e.g. chewing gum.
- Something for your hands to fiddle with, e.g. a toy or worry beads.
- Nicotine chewing gum or patches, but do follow the instructions on the package.
- Professional help from a doctor, an acupuncturist or a hypnotist.
- Taking vitamin C, fruit or fruit juice to help the body rid itself of nicotine more quickly.
- Taking a homeopathic medicine, see page 85.

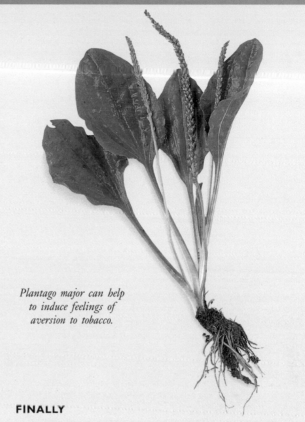

Plantago major can help to induce feelings of aversion to tobacco.

FINALLY

- Decide the best day for you to quit: you may prefer to be busy or to be relaxed, or even on vacation away from your normal routine.
- Ask your family and friends for support.

GIVING UP

THE DAY BEFORE:

- Review your plans.
- Get rid of ashtrays, lighters and cigarettes.

THE DAY AND AFTER:

- Just take one day at a time, do not think too much about the future.
- When tempted to smoke, do something else, don't just sit and think about it. Carefully read through your plans again.
- Remember that anyone who says, 'Go on, just have one cigarette' is probably jealous: many surveys have shown that the majority of smokers would prefer to be ex-smokers like you.
- Be patient; remember the craving will go away.

Angina
Heart or chest pain

Angina occurs because the arteries taking blood to the heart muscle cannot supply the amount of blood it requires to function normally. When this occurs, chest pain may be experienced. The pain does not normally occur at rest; more often it is felt when there is increased activity by the heart, such as during exercise, or with anemia and obesity. Angina can occur in virtually any adult age group, but people over 45 are those most commonly affected.

The chest pain is described as a tightness or feeling of constriction, and in about half the patients pain will radiate down one or both arms and occasionally to the throat or jaw. The arm pain is often described as a numbness. Typically, the pain is related to exertion, a heavy meal or excitement. It usually passes off after a few minutes' rest, but if it continues, a heart attack may have occurred. Well over half of angina sufferers have shortness of breath and raised blood pressure. Anxiety, inflammation of the esophagus and gall bladder, and peptic ulceration can all produce similar pains so it is important to consult your doctor for a diagnosis. ***Always consult your doctor if chest pain develops for no obvious reason.***

SYMPTOMS / MEDICINE

Symptoms	Medicine
❧ Extreme anxiety and fear, with palpitations and intense pain in the region of the heart. ❧ Pain also radiates down the left arm, with numbness occurring in the fingers.	⊛ Aconitum napellus
❧ Pain radiates to the region of the left elbow.	⊛ Arnica montana
❧ Chest feels as if it is constricted by an iron band. ❧ A suffocating feeling with a cold sweat.	⊛ Cactus grandiflorus
❧ Angina pains with associated asthma and muscle cramps.	⊛ Cuprum metallicum
❧ Pain radiates from the back of the breastbone to the arms. ❧ Much gas and labored breathing.	⊛ Dioscorea villosa
❧ Slightest exertion brings on the angina. ❧ Palpitations and shortness of breath may also be present.	⊛ Glonoinum
❧ Violent cramping pain extending to the armpit and down the arm to the fingers, with a numb sensation in the arm.	⊛ Latrodectus mactans
❧ Chest pain with pain in the right arm.	⊛ Lilium tigrinum
❧ Constricting pains around heart.	⊛ Magnesia phosphorica
❧ Pain extends to the nape of the neck, left shoulder and arm. ❧ Great anxiety and fear of death.	⊛ Naja tripudians
❧ Pain is sharp and lancing. ❧ Angina alternates with voice loss.	⊛ Oxalicum acidum
❧ A drink of hot water relieves the pain, which is violent and greatly aggravated by motion.	⊛ Spigelia anthelmia
❧ Pain accompanied by faintness, suffocation and an anxious sweat, comes on after midnight.	⊛ Spongia tosta
❧ Pain is over the heart, radiating in all directions. ❧ Pain and shortness of breath that is worse when lying on the left side.	⊛ Tabacum

DOSAGE

USE THE 30C POTENCY. TAKE IMMEDIATELY THE SYMPTOMS OCCUR AND REPEAT EVERY 20 MINUTES UNTIL AN IMPROVEMENT IS NOTED. THEN TAKE AT INCREASING INTERVALS, IF NECESSARY.

Anemia

This is a condition in which the red cells of the blood fail to carry enough oxygen for the body's needs. *You should consult your doctor if you think you are anemic because the underlying cause needs to be diagnosed.* The most common type of anemia in women is caused by iron deficiency as a result of iron being lost, during heavy periods or as a result of pregnancy, more quickly than it can be replaced by the diet. The medicines below can be taken in addition to conventional treatment, if this is prescribed.

DOSAGE

USE THE 12C POTENCY. TAKE TWICE A DAY FOR UP TO TWO WEEKS.

SYMPTOMS / MEDICINE

Symptoms	Medicine
➼ Exhaustion following blood loss. ➼ Sensitivity to cold.	⊛ Chinchona officinalis
➼ Weakness and lassitude. ➼ Visual disturbance.	⊛ Cyclamen europaeum
➼ If pale but with a tendency to flush easily.	⊛ Ferrum metallicum
➼ If all the symptoms are better when lying down.	⊛ Manganum aceticum
➼ Exhaustion following loss of blood. ➼ Symptoms are generally aggravated by heat.	⊛ Natrum muriaticum

Fluid retention
Edema

Swelling of the body due to fluid retention can have several causes. It can occur in diseases of the heart, the liver, the lungs and the kidneys, and if any of these are suspected, a doctor should be consulted. It also develops through protein deficiency during periods of famine and starvation. However, swelling of the feet and ankles may occur in normal adults if they stand for too long, or sit for long periods in cramped conditions, such as in an airplane. It frequently occurs in middle age if you are overweight. *Fluid retention during a pregnancy may be an indication of pre-eclampsia, so if it occurs, your doctor or midwife should be consulted.*

SYMPTOMS / MEDICINE

Symptoms	Medicine
➼ Skin becomes waxy in color and to the touch. ➼ Great thirst, invariably with stomach upsets.	⊛ Aceticum acidum
➼ A transparent and waxy-looking skin. ➼ No thirst. ➼ Urine is scanty and may contain a dark deposit.	⊛ Apis mellifica
➼ Feelings of great thirst but drinking upsets the stomach. ➼ A feeling of pressure in the chest and in the abdomen. ➼ Frequent indigestion.	⊛ Apocynum cannabinum
➼ Great thirst but only for small amounts of fluid, taken very frequently. ➼ A shortness of breath on exertion, but it may also disturb sleep.	⊛ Arsenicum album

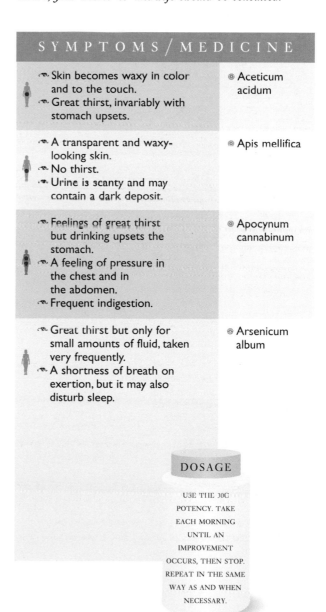

DOSAGE

USE THE 30C POTENCY. TAKE EACH MORNING UNTIL AN IMPROVEMENT OCCURS, THEN STOP. REPEAT IN THE SAME WAY AS AND WHEN NECESSARY.

High blood pressure

Hypertension

Initial diagnosis and investigation of this condition should be made by a doctor. Homeopathic treatment may be possible, but this should always be administered under medical supervision. There are several causes of high blood pressure, including being overweight and drinking too much alcohol, but often no cause is found. If this is the case patients are said to have essential hypertension. Symptoms may be absent, but some patients complain of dizziness, tinnitus (noises in the ear) and headache. Nosebleeds probably occur more often than in people with normal blood pressure.

SYMPTOMS / MEDICINE

Symptoms	Medicine
❧ Pain occurs behind the breastbone at night. ❧ Very despondent and may even feel suicidal. ❧ Signs of hardening of the arteries may be present such as angina, dizziness and vertigo.	◉ Aurum metallicum
❧ Blood pressure may be very high. ❧ Palpitations are also present, which become worse when lying on the left side. ❧ Pulse is full and hard.	◉ Baryta carbonica
❧ Violent, irregular palpitations, with a headache that is worse for noise and smell. ❧ Insomnia.	◉ Coffea cruda
❧ Nose feels very blocked and swollen. ❧ Palpitations occur from the least exertion. ❧ Anxiety and depression complicate illness.	◉ Iodium
❧ Raised blood pressure which comes about at the menopause. ❧ Headaches, fainting and flushing. ❧ Heart feels too large and there is a cramp-like pain in the chest wall over the heart.	◉ Lachesis mutus
❧ Heart rate is very rapid, with pain over the heart area. ❧ There is also asthma of cardiac origin and rheumatism. ❧ Pulse becomes weak and irregular. ❧ Nosebleeds and frontal headaches.	◉ Lycopus virginicus
❧ A rapid, irregular heart rate with angina. ❧ There is also a profuse flow of urine. ❧ Excessive gas.	◉ Cystisus scoparius
❧ Face becomes flushed easily. ❧ A strong arterial pulse. ❧ Vertigo with headache and nausea.	◉ Strontium carbonicum
❧ Pulse is slow, soft, weak and irregular. ❧ Constant burning pain over the heart. ❧ Face is flushed and congested and feels quite quarrelsome.	◉ Veratrum viride

DOSAGE

USE THE 30C POTENCY. TAKE TWICE A DAY. FREQUENT BLOOD–PRESSURE READINGS AND REASSESSMENT SHOULD BE MADE AND THE TREATMENT CHANGED OR MODIFIED, IF NECESSARY.

Varicose veins and phlebitis

*V*eins that become tortuous and distended are said to be varicose (the word itself means swollen and knotted). Pregnancy is one of the most common causes of varicose veins, but they may also be caused by constipation, prolonged standing and excess weight. Varicose veins may become painful and the skin can show discoloration, especially around the lower part of the leg. Swelling of the ankles is another feature and this is frequently the result of prolonged standing.

Once a vein becomes varicose, it may get worse and can never become a normal vein again as the elasticity of the vein wall has been destroyed.

A common complication of varicose veins is phlebitis – inflammation of the vein. The area affected is red, hot and painful. This usually takes place in a vein on the surface of the leg and is reasonably easy to treat with local compresses and the appropriate homeopathic medicine. *If, however, one of the deeper leg veins is inflamed and clotted (known as deep vein thrombosis or DVT), it becomes swollen and very painful. Deep vein thrombosis is a serious condition which needs urgent medical help to treat it.*

DOSAGE

USE THE 12C POTENCY. TAKE TWICE A DAY UNTIL AN IMPROVEMENT OCCURS. REPEAT IF SYMPTOMS RETURN.

SYMPTOMS / MEDICINE

Symptoms	Medicine
Varicose veins that are bruised and sore. Walking is difficult.	Bellis perennis
Specifically for varicose veins and enlarged, prominent veins that are worse during rest but better for warm applications.	Calcarea fluorica
Veins are distended and itch, especially in the evening and in bed.	Carbo vegetabilis
Varicose veins, often with small areas of 'spider veins'.	Hydrofluoricum acidum
Affected area feels bruised and sore. Inflammation of the veins (phlebitis).	Hamamelis virginiana
Painful varicose veins occurring in pregnancy.	Millefolium
Varicose veins with acute phlebitis. Veins are swollen, sensitive and feel as if they will burst unless the leg is elevated.	Vipera berus
Large veins, with sweaty and restless feet.	Zincum metallicum

Palpitations

*T*he normal resting adult heart beats regularly at an average rate of 60 times per minute and is governed by the speed of electrical signals originating from the natural pacemaker of the heart. Palpitations are unpleasant sensations of irregular and/or forceful beating. In many patients with palpitations no heart disease or abnormal heart rhythms can be found and the reason for their palpitations is unknown although anxiety is often one of the causes. ***Consult a doctor.***

SYMPTOMS / MEDICINE	
Palpitations with burning and distension of the stomach and abdomen.	◉ Abies canadensis
Palpitations with anxiety, fainting and tingling fingers.	◉ Aconitum napellus
Palpitations with pain over the heart and shortness of breath.	◉ Adonis vernalis
Violent palpitations accompanied by vertigo, headache and restlessness.	◉ Aethusa cynapium
Irregular, violent palpitations after smoking.	◉ Agaricus muscarius
Palpitations are felt with a feeling of a lump in the chest and that are worse in the open air. Pale face.	◉ Ambra grisea
Wakes up with palpitations accompanied by fear, cold sweat, loud and difficult breathing and trembling hands.	◉ Ammonium carbonicum
Frequent headaches and palpitations.	◉ Amyl nitrosum
Palpitations in the elderly.	◉ Anacardium orientale
Palpitations that are worse when lying on the right side.	◉ Argentum nitricum
Pulse is more rapid in the morning.	◉ Arsenicum album
Violent, throbbing palpitations from exertion.	◉ Belladonna
Violent palpitations that are worse when lying on the left side. Palpitations just before a period.	◉ Cactus grandiflorus
Slightest emotion causes palpitations. Palpitations in overweight women.	◉ Calcarea arsenicosa
Palpitations that happen at night and after eating.	◉ Calcarea arsenicica
Nervous palpitations, especially after excessive excitement.	◉ Coffea cruda
Palpitations that come with menstruation.	◉ Crotalus horridus
Palpitations that occur from the slightest movement.	◉ Digitalis purpurea
Palpitations that happen after the slightest exertion, or when laughing or coughing, and which are accompanied by vertigo.	◉ Iberis amara

DOSAGE

USE THE 12C POTENCY. TAKE EVERY 20 MINUTES UNTIL AN IMPROVEMENT IS MAINTAINED.

☙ Palpitations with a burning sensation in the heart region.	◉ Kali carbonicum
☙ Palpitations that are worse when bending forward.	◉ Kalmia latifolia
☙ Palpitations accompanied by fainting during menstruation.	◉ Lachesis mutus
☙ Palpitations during the night, lying on the left side or at about 4 am.	◉ Lycopodium clavatum
☙ Palpitations that come about from nervous irritation.	◉ Lycopus virginicus
☙ Palpitations while sitting, and which are better for moving about.	◉ Magnesia muriatica
☙ A fluttering, palpitating heart, often with heartburn.	◉ Natrum muriaticum
☙ Palpitations and shortness of breath in heart disease, worse for thinking about them.	◉ Oxalicum acidum
☙ Violent palpitations that come with anxiety when lying on the left side.	◉ Phosphorus
☙ Palpitations and trembling that occur while sitting still.	◉ Rhus toxicodendron
☙ Palpitations with contracted, intermittent pulse.	◉ Secale cornutum
☙ Violent and intermittent palpitations.	◉ Sepia
☙ Frequent bouts of palpitations occur, accompanied by a foul mouth odor.	◉ Spigelia anthelmia
☙ Palpitations just before menstruation.	◉ Spongia tosta
☙ Anemia is accompanied by palpitations and breathlessness.	◉ Strophanthus hispidus
☙ Palpitations that occur when lying on the left side.	◉ Tabacum
☙ Palpitations with anxiety and noisy breathing.	◉ Veratrum album
☙ Difficult breathing, anxiety and palpitations. Feelings are out of control.	◉ Viola odorata
☙ Palpitations during lovemaking.	◉ Viscum album

Bronchitis

*A*cute bronchitis occurs when the mucous membranes that line the bronchi and bronchioles become inflamed, usually as a result of a viral infection. In chronic bronchitis, the inflammation is more or less permanent, but the symptoms can be made worse by infection. Chronic bronchitis is nearly always because of years of smoking or exposure to air pollution. *Bronchitis should be diagnosed and treated by a doctor, but you may find homeopathic medicines provide additional symptom relief.* See also Asthma, page 84.

DOSAGE

USE THE 12C POTENCY. FOR ACUTE BRONCHITIS TAKE FOUR TIMES A DAY FOR UP TO FOUR DAYS. FOR CHRONIC BRONCHITIS TAKE TWICE A DAY ON TWO DAYS EACH WEEK WHEN SYMPTOMS ARE PRESENT

SYMPTOMS / MEDICINE

☙ Coarse rattling in the chest or larynx. ☙ Cough sounds 'wet' but little phlegm is coughed up. ☙ Feeling of suffocation.	◉ Antimonium tartaricum
☙ A dry and painful cough with need to hold the chest while coughing. ☙ A desire to be left alone and to keep still. ☙ Great thirst and a preference for large drinks.	◉ Bryonia
☙ A rattling cough and a feeling of suffocation. ☙ Phlegm may be bloodstained. ☙ There is associated nausea.	◉ Ipecacuanha
☙ Stringy phlegm, often yellow, which is difficult to cough up. ☙ Cough is worse after waking and after eating. ☙ Symptoms are worse around 4–5 am.	◉ Kali bichromicum
☙ Breathing is difficult, and worse lying flat, but better when sitting up and leaning forward. ☙ Symptoms are worse at 2–4 am. ☙ Thick, foul-tasting phlegm.	◉ Kali carbonicum
☙ Recurrent colds that keep going to the chest. ☙ A lingering tickly cough is aggravated by cold air, exertion and lying flat. ☙ Craves ice-cold drinks.	◉ Phosphorus

Asthma

The main symptoms of asthma are wheezing and breathlessness, which are caused when the respiratory tubes called the bronchi go into spasm. They may be associated with a chest infection, but they can also be brought on by allergy, exercise, stress and psychological factors. Asthma is a serious condition that can occur at any age and, occasionally, can be fatal. *Medical help is needed if there is no quick response to homeopathic home treatment.* The following medicines may be of help during an acute attack. For the correct overall management of asthma, a deeper constitutional treatment from a homeopathic doctor is required – generally during a dormant phase of the illness.

SYMPTOMS / MEDICINE

Symptoms	Medicine
❧ A sudden violent attack after exposure to cold, dry winds. ❧ Very restless, frightened and anxious. ❧ A hoarse, dry, croupy cough with breathlessness with the slightest movement.	⊛ Aconitum napellus
❧ Extreme wheeziness exists with shortness of breath and much mucus. ❧ Increasingly weak, drowsy and sweaty. ❧ Help may be needed to sit up to breathe and cough up mucus. ❧ Pale and irritable but not thirsty.	⊛ Antimonium tartaricum *plus urgent medical attention*
❧ Cough is worse for lying down. ❧ Attack comes in the middle of the night. ❧ Frequent sneezing. ❧ Feeling of something in the throat.	⊛ Aralia racemosa
❧ Attacks between midnight and 3 am. ❧ Restless and fears death by suffocation. ❧ Attack is better for bending forward, for warmth applied to the chest and from warm drinks. ❧ Worse in the cold air.	⊛ Arsenicum album
❧ Attacks alternate with vomiting. ❧ Suffocative attacks beginning around 3 am. ❧ Face goes blue with coughing.	⊛ Cuprum metallicum *plus urgent medical attention*
❧ A sudden onset of wheezing that is worse from movement. ❧ Anxiety and a sensation of weight on the chest. ❧ A constant, non-productive cough that causes gagging and/or vomiting. ❧ Cold sweats.	⊛ Ipecacuanha *plus urgent medical attention*
❧ Attack starts between 3 and 4 am. ❧ Attack is better for sitting up and leaning forward. ❧ Stringy yellow mucus. ❧ Asthma is worse at 3 am and is better for leaning forward.	⊛ Kali bichromicum
❧ Asthma comes on with hay fever and spasms of sneezing.	⊛ Lachesis mutus
❧ Worse in damp weather and often accompanies hay fever. ❧ Attacks start around 4–5 am with a productive cough and copious sputum. ❧ Sitting up and holding chest eases breathing.	⊛ Natrum sulphuricum
❧ Wakes around midnight with a laryngeal cough and feeling of suffocation. ❧ Nose is blocked so breathes through mouth.	⊛ Sambucus nigra *plus urgent medical attention*

DOSAGE

USE THE 30C POTENCY. TAKE EVERY 15 MINUTES UNTIL THERE IS AN IMPROVEMENT. THEN TAKE AT INCREASING INTERVALS AS AND WHEN NECESSARY. IF THERE IS NO QUICK RESPONSE, SEEK MEDICAL HELP.

Giving up smoking

Smoking is an addiction which many people find very hard to give up. A few facts about it may help . . .

❧ Smoking is responsible for many thousands of deaths each year and smokers have a two in five risk of dying before the age of 65.

❧ Smokers are twice as likely to die of heart disease as non-smokers.

❧ 95 per cent of people who suffer from bronchitis are regular smokers.

❧ 90 per cent of deaths that occur from lung cancer are smoking related.

❧ Strokes happen 70 per cent more frequently in smokers than non-smokers.

❧ 95 per cent of people who suffer from leg artery disease are smokers.

❧ Smoking during pregnancy leads to low birth-weight babies and has recently been implicated in sudden crib death syndrome.

The most important feature in giving up smoking is the resolve of the smoker. Homeopathy can help, but will-power and determination are also vital. There are several medicines that are helpful for the symptoms that are caused by tobacco abuse, but one of the following four homeopathic medicines may be tried to overcome the addiction.

SYMPTOMS / MEDICINE	
❧ Modifies the craving of tobacco	❂ Caladium seguinum
❧ May induce an aversion to tobacco.	❂ Plantago major
❧ Where there is suppresssed anger and resentment.	❂ Staphysagria
❧ Relieves the craving for tobacco.	❂ Tabacum

DOSAGE

USE THE 12C POTENCY. TAKE THREE TIMES A DAY UNTIL THE HABIT HAS BEEN OVERCOME.

Cough

A cough occurs as a response to an irritant, such as mucus, phlegm, dust or smoke, either in the throat or in the airway. Coughing is commonly the result of a viral infection, such as a cold. *If you have a high temperature, weight loss or if your cough persists for more than a week or two you should consult your doctor.*

SYMPTOMS / MEDICINE	
❧ A hard dry cough caused by exposure to a cold wind or after a fright.	❂ Aconitum napellus
❧ For when the mucus is noisy but not coughed up. ❧ When the cough is relieved by sitting up.	❂ Antimonium tartaricum
❧ A dry painful cough, that is worse in a warm room.	❂ Bryonia
❧ A dry, tickling cough that is relieved by a cold drink. ❧ Cough may cause slight incontinence.	❂ Causticum
❧ Paroxysmal coughing, often caused by thick sticky mucus in the throat.	❂ Coccus cacti
❧ A gurgling but spasmodic cough. ❧ Cough is relieved by a cold drink.	❂ Cuprum metallicum
❧ Long periods of rapid, barking choking cough. ❧ Cough is often caused by lying down.	❂ Drosera rotundifolia
❧ A barking cough with yellow, stringy phlegm.	❂ Kali bichromicum
❧ A tickling dry cough is aggravated by cold air.	❂ Rumex crispus
❧ A hollow, barking cough that is worse in a warm room. ❧ Cough is relieved by warm food and drink.	❂ Spongia tosta

DOSAGE

USE THE 12C POTENCY. REPEAT EVERY 30 MINUTES IF NECESSARY.

CHAPTER 6

THE DIGESTIVE SYSTEM

IF YOU LIVE for 70 years, your digestive system will have processed about 100 tons of food, absorbing the nutrients and discharging the residue. This enormous task takes place within the digestive or alimentary canal. Essentially, this is a tube, about 9m/30ft in length, that starts at the mouth and then continues through the esophagus, the stomach, the small and large intestines, the rectum and ends at the anus. The other organs of digestion are the salivary glands, the liver and the pancreas.

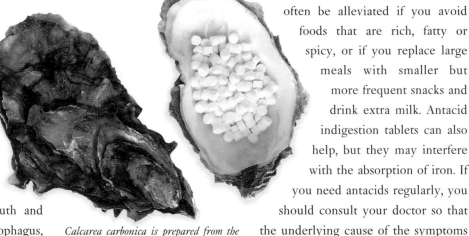

Calcarea carbonica is prepared from the middle layer of the shell of an oyster.

For your food to be of use to your body it has to be broken down physically, by being chewed in the mouth and churned in the stomach, and chemically, by the digestive juices. These juices are secreted by the salivary glands, by glands within the walls of the stomach and small intestine, and by the liver and pancreas.

The lining of the small intestine is constructed with numerous folds and microscopic projections, and has been estimated to be the size of a tennis court. This huge area is available to enable the nutrients from the liquid products of digestion to be absorbed into the bloodstream. The residue passes into the large intestine, where much of the remaining liquid is taken into the body and the solid is discharged through the anus, as stools or feces.

INDIGESTION

Eating can cause a number of symptoms, such as pain in the upper abdomen or behind the breastbone (heartburn), nausea and burping (gas). These symptoms can

Graphite is the naturally occurring mineral used in lead pencils and also in the preparation of the medicine Graphites.

often be alleviated if you avoid foods that are rich, fatty or spicy, or if you replace large meals with smaller but more frequent snacks and drink extra milk. Antacid indigestion tablets can also help, but they may interfere with the absorption of iron. If you need antacids regularly, you should consult your doctor so that the underlying cause of the symptoms can be investigated.

Indigestion can be a particular problem in pregnancy because of hormonal changes and because, in late pregnancy, the baby presses onto the stomach.

CONSTIPATION

Infrequency of bowel action often causes unnecessary anxiety as it is not unhealthy to have a bowel action only twice a week if the stool is soft. The symptoms of constipation are infrequent, hard stools that are painful to pass and may cause bleeding from the anus.

If you do have a tendency to constipation, it may help to eat a diet that is higher in fiber (see page 88). Try eating more fruit and vegetables, beans, and wholegrains, such as brown rice and wholewheat flour or bread. If you have been used to white flour and grains, you should change your diet gradually so that you give your digestion enough time to adapt to the different foods that you are eating. Try to drink at least 2 litres/3 pints of liquid per day, and more in hot weather or when you are in a hot climate. **You should always consult your doctor rightaway if you suddenly become constipated for no apparent reason.**

GUT FEELINGS

People will often be sick at the side of the road after a traffic accident. This is part of the well-known 'fight or flight' reaction when the body produces a surge of adrenalin in response to shock and sudden fear. When your life is put at risk certain functions that are not immediately essential, such as the digestion of food, are put on hold, and this sometimes causes the contents of the stomach and bowel to be ejected.

Diarrhea before a public performance or important interview is another example of the same process. It is hardly surprising, therefore, to find that lesser but perhaps more relentless stresses can affect the activity of the digestive system. Doctors have long recognized that altered appetite, indigestion and the symptoms of irritable bowel syndrome (see box on page 89) are often made worse by worry and anxiety. Homeopathy can do much to relieve the symptoms of such digestive system disorders, both as symptom medicines and on a more constitutional basis. *If, with self-medication, your symptoms do not respond within a couple of weeks, you should consult your doctor to check the diagnosis. Complete loss of appetite, unexplained weight loss and difficult or painful swallowing require an urgent medical opinion.*

GASTROENTERITIS

Gastroenteritis is the inflammation of the stomach and intestines that can follow various infections, dietary indiscretions, such as too much alcohol or spicy food, or certain drugs, including antibiotics. Symptoms include pain, vomiting and diarrhea, and homeopathic medicines can be very helpful in easing the discomfort.

Medical advice is needed if your symptoms are severe, last longer than 48 hours, if you are feverish, or if there is blood in the stools.

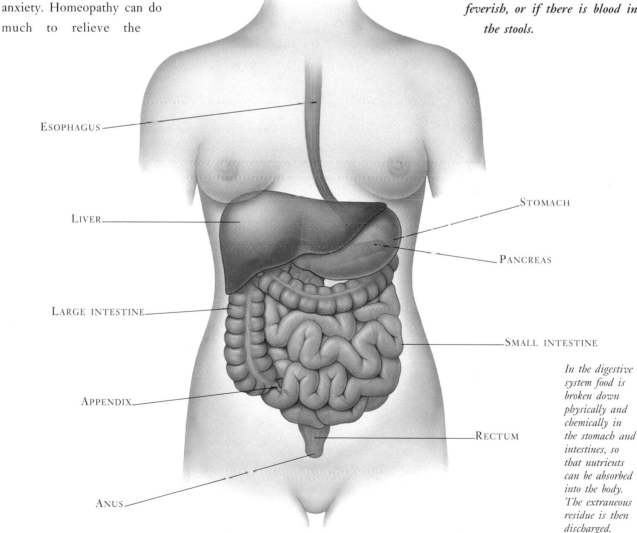

ESOPHAGUS

LIVER

LARGE INTESTINE

APPENDIX

ANUS

STOMACH

PANCREAS

SMALL INTESTINE

RECTUM

In the digestive system food is broken down physically and chemically in the stomach and intestines, so that nutrients can be absorbed into the body. The extraneous residue is then discharged.

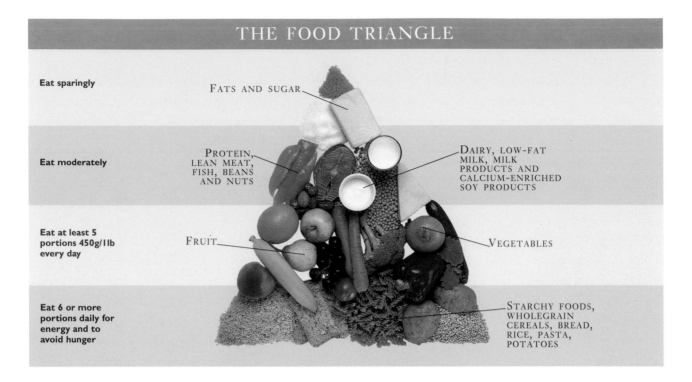

THE FOOD TRIANGLE

Eat sparingly

FATS AND SUGAR

Eat moderately

PROTEIN, LEAN MEAT, FISH, BEANS AND NUTS

DAIRY, LOW-FAT MILK, MILK PRODUCTS AND CALCIUM-ENRICHED SOY PRODUCTS

Eat at least 5 portions 450g/1lb every day

FRUIT

VEGETABLES

Eat 6 or more portions daily for energy and to avoid hunger

STARCHY FOODS, WHOLEGRAIN CEREALS, BREAD, RICE, PASTA, POTATOES

More serious causes of diarrhea, such as ulcerative colitis and Crohn's disease, can often be helped by homeopathy but medical supervision is essential.

EAT FOR HEALTH

The father of modern homeopathy, Samuel Hahnemann (see page 10), considered that ill health caused by malnutrition was not 'true disease' and he was one of the earliest doctors to advocate a nutritious diet. If he were alive today, he would be amazed at the current view that malnutrition in Western countries more often results from eating the wrong foods rather than having too little food.

Recent research has implicated the modern Western diet as being among the main causes of heart disease and cancer: these are, of course, 'true diseases', but is is thought that they can often be avoided or at least postponed by eating a healthy diet. Unfortunately, as each new item of research hits the headlines it often contradicts previous press reports and medical advice, and there is much public confusion about what a healthy diet really is.

Most experts now accept that in developed countries people eat too much fat, particularly the saturated fat from animal sources, and too little fresh fruit and vegetables. Your can limit your animal fats by cutting obvious fat off meat and eating low-fat dairy products. Remember there are also hidden animal fats in biscuits, cakes and chocolate.

The current recommendations for a diet that will contain all the different foods that you need each day are indicated in the 'food triangle' above.

SOME HIGH-FIBRE FOODS

food	grams of fibre per 100gm/4oz
Kidney beans, dried	.28
Dried apricots, uncooked	.27
Dried figs, uncooked	.21
Almonds, shelled	.16
Crispbreads	.13
Lentils, dried	.12
Wholewheat flour	.11
Wholewheat pasta, dried	.11
Brazil nuts, shelled	.10
Brown rice	.5
Leafy greens, boiled	.4
Carrots	.4
Baked potato with skin	.3

IRRITABLE BOWEL SYNDROME

Irritable bowel syndrome (IBS), also known as spastic or irritable colon, usually starts in the early to mid adult years. Once you have it, the condition tends to come and go throughout your life.

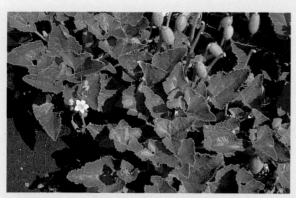

Colocynthis derived from the plant, Citrullus colocynthis, often soothes uncomfortable, colicky pains, such as those that occur during an attack of irritable bowel syndrome.

WHAT IS IT?

IBS is a disturbance of the action of the muscles in the walls of the large bowel that propel the residue from the digestive system towards the rectum. Before the diagnosis can be made it is essential that your doctor excludes other diseases.

WHAT ARE THE SYMPTOMS?

- Intermittent, cramping abdominal pain.
- Irregular bowel habit i.e. constipation, diarrhea or bouts of both.
- Abdominal distension (swelling), usually on the left side that is relieved by a bowel movement or by passing gas.
- Excessive gas in the bowel with rumbles and gurgles.
- A sense of incomplete evacuation after a bowel movement.
- Eating often makes the symptoms worse.

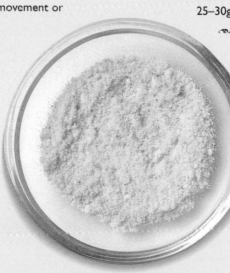

Suphur may help to ease irritable bowel syndrome when there is diarrhea that occurs about 5 am.

WHAT ARE THE CAUSES?

The causes of IBS are not fully understood, but they appear to be related to, or at least made worse by, stress. Many doctors believe that there are also dietary causes involved.

SELF-HELP

1 REDUCE STRESS

- Think about changes in your lifestyle that would reduce your stress levels. Take time off work regularly to relax. Have at least one vacation a year.
- Take more exercise. This helps to burn up the adrenalin produced by the anxieties and frustrations of life. Exercise also benefits your heart and bones.
- Learn relaxation techniques. Sign up for a class in relaxation, meditation or yoga. Treat yourself to a massage or aromatherapy: if you can't afford to go to an expert, get a self-help book from the library and experiment with your partner or a friend.
- Adopt a positive approach to your life. Go to self-assertion classes. Do something about the office bully or anything else that is upsetting you.

2 CHANGE YOUR DIET

Make changes to your diet gradually. Dramatic changes in your eating habits tend to upset the digestive system. There is no single change that will benefit everyone: so be prepared to spend some time finding out what really suits you best.

- Try eating more fiber: you should eat 25–30gm/⅔–1oz of fiber a day (see left).
- Eat less sugar, including honey. If you crave a sweet snack, choose dried fruit (this will also increase your fiber intake).
- Some people are helped by eating less fat, drinking more water, or by eating smaller meals more frequently.
- Keep a food and symptom diary for a few weeks: this may help to suggest foods that are causing the problematic symptoms.

Belching and gas

*T*he sudden expulsion of gas from the stomach through the mouth known as belching often occurs after eating certain foods, especially highly seasoned foods, peas and beans, some vegetables and fruit that have a high carbohydrate content. Flatulence is also often present with digestive upsets, such as indigestion or when you suffer from a stomach problem and diarrhea. It can also be a problem if you have swallowed excess air when you are rushing and have eaten a meal too quickly.

SYMPTOMS/MEDICINE

Symptoms	Medicine
↝ Sour belching with vomiting. ↝ Violent stomach pain. ↝ A cold sweat and cold skin.	⊛ Aceticum acidum
↝ Loss of appetite. ↝ A craving for acidic foods. ↝ The belch tastes of the food just eaten.	⊛ Antimonium crudum
↝ Belching accompanies stomach upsets. ↝ Pain over stomach, which radiates to all parts of the abdomen.	⊛ Argentum nitricum
↝ Belching, heaviness, fullness and sleepiness occur together ↝ Belching is worse when lying down.	⊛ Carbo vegetabilis
↝ Much flatulence that is not relieved from bitter regurgitation. ↝ Belching is worse after eating fruit.	⊛ Chinchona officinalis
↝ Large quantities of offensive gas are belched.	⊛ Dioscorea villosa
↝ A burning sensation in the pharynx. ↝ Food tastes sour. ↝ Abdomen is bloated.	⊛ Lycopodium clavatum
↝ Flatulent colic accompanied by belching of gas. ↝ Bending double provides relief.	⊛ Magnesia phosphorica
↝ Chronic indigestion. ↝ Frequent belching. ↝ Sour stomach.	⊛ Natrum carbonicum
↝ Sour, bitter difficult belches.	⊛ Nux vomica
↝ Belches large quantities of gas straight after eating.	⊛ Phosphorus
↝ Hot, sour belching.	⊛ Podophyllum
↝ Belching alternates with hiccoughs.	⊛ Wyethia helenioides

DOSAGE

USE THE 30C POTENCY. TAKE THREE TIMES A DAY FOR TWO TO THREE DAYS.

Constipation

Constipation is a condition where the bowels move only infrequently and with difficulty. Most cases arise from a poor diet, where too much refined food, such as white bread and cakes is eaten. An increased intake of fiber in the form of fruit and vegetables, bran, wholewheat bread and brown rice will often relieve the condition. Unfortunately, constipation is a common occurrence during pregnancy where it then tends to aggravate piles or hemorrhoids and varicose veins, if they are present. It is also one of the symptoms of Irritable bowel syndrome, see page 89.

SYMPTOMS / MEDICINE

Symptoms	Medicine
~ Stools are either soft and sticky, or hard and dry. ~ Defecation is difficult and there is no desire to move the bowels. ~ Even a soft stool requires considerable straining.	Alumina
~ Stools are hard, dry, dark and lumpy. ~ Defecation is difficult because of a lack of urge.	Bryonia
~ Stools are smelly, large and lumpy and stuck together with mucus. ~ Stools are painful to pass and causes a smarting, sore anal pain.	Graphites
~ Hard, dry stools which are painful to pass. ~ Ineffectual urging, with the rectum protruding. ~ Piles or hemorrhoids frequently develop.	Lycopodium clavatum
~ Frequent ineffectual desire. ~ Incomplete stools, so the rectum feels unemptied. ~ Laxatives may have been taken for a long time.	Nux vomica
~ A complete lack of desire to pass stools. ~ Stool is composed of hard little balls which protrude and then recede. ~ Constipation affects the appetite, which is poor.	Opium *(prescription required in USA)*
~ Frequent, unsuccessful urging. ~ Stools seem to adhere to the rectum like soft clay. ~ Often helpful if other homeopathic medicines fail.	Platinum metallicum
~ Stools are hard, dry, lumpy and black, and may become impacted. ~ Rectum seems paralyzed. ~ Anus is in spasm and this produces great pain.	Plumbum metallicum
~ Stools are hard, in balls and are difficult to pass. ~ Rectal pain during and after stools are passed.	Sepia
~ A hard stool is felt which may slip back when partially expelled.	Silicea
~ Stools are hard, dry, black and smelly. ~ Anal irritation. ~ Pain and burning with defecation. ~ Reluctance to defecate because of the pain.	Sulphur

DOSAGE

USE THE 6C POTENCY. TAKE THREE TIMES A DAY UNTIL AN IMPROVEMENT OCCURS, THEN REDUCE TO TWICE A DAY FOR THREE DAYS, ONCE A DAY FOR THREE DAYS, THEN STOP.

Indigestion and heartburn

*I*ndigestion is the discomfort that is felt in the upper abdomen which usually occurs after eating too much food, eating too quickly or after eating fatty or highly spiced foods. Emotional stress can also be a factor. However, the term indigestion is often also used to describe a variety of symptoms including belching (see page 90), nausea and vomiting (see page 94) and also heartburn.

Heartburn is a burning pain behind the breastbone that can be caused by the backflow of stomach acid during pregnancy, a hiatus hernia (protrusion of part of the stomach into the chest) or obesity. It is aggravated by lying flat, by bending over and by drinking alcohol. (See also Peptic ulcers, page 93.) *If you have regular bouts of indigestion, you should see your doctor so that the underlying cause can be investigated.*

SYMPTOMS / MEDICINE

Symptoms	Medicine
Indigestion from stress and tension. No food is desired. Vomiting is also usually present.	Aletris farinosa
Pain in the pit of the stomach. Heartburn and nausea, with belching. Chilliness.	Ammonium carbonicum
Nervous indigestion is relieved by food.	Anacardium orientale
Indigestion after eating fruit, acidic foods, ice cream or cold drinks.	Arsenicum album
Indigestion after drinking cold drinks taken when you are overheated.	Bryonia
Heartburn with loud belching. Craving for indigestible things.	Calcarea carbonica
Flatulent indigestion. Craving for stimulants such as coffee. A sinking feeling in the pit of the stomach. Great thirst.	Capsicum annuum
Nausea, acrid heartburn and acid belching. Indigestion is worse after going to bed and lying down. Eating relieves the indigestion temporarily.	Conium maculatum
Food tastes sour. Distension and indigestion from eating carbohydrates. Excessive hunger but the stomach feels full after eating only a small amount of food.	Lycopodium clavatum
Thirst for cold drinks. Continual hunger. Hiccoughs and acid regurgitation.	Mercurius solubilis
Heartburn with palpitations.	Natrum muriaticum
Sour belches and taste. A yellow-creamy coating appears on the tongue.	Natrum phosphoricum
Depression. Immense hunger and craving for fats and salt.	Nitricum acidum
Flatulent indigestion with hiccoughs.	Nux moschata

❧ Ravenous appetite for foods that disagree, as well as highly seasoned foods and coffee.	◉ Nux vomica
❧ Acid indigestion. ❧ Abdomen feels bloated. ❧ Nausea at the sight or smell of food. ❧ A faint, sinking feeling that is not eased by eating.	◉ Sepia
❧ Great acidity with either a complete loss of, or excessive, appetite. ❧ Milk disagrees with the digestive system. ❧ Feels weak and faint at around 11 am.	◉ Sulphur
❧ Heartburn from eating sweet things.	◉ Zincum metallicum

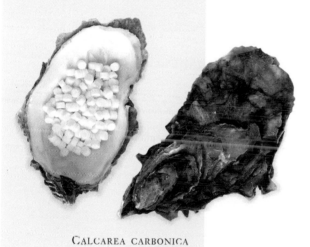

CALCAREA CARBONICA

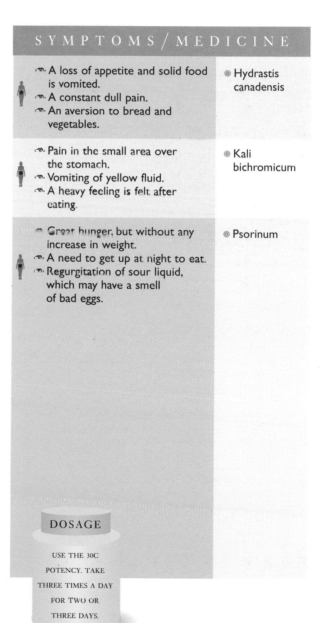DOSAGE

USE THE 12C POTENCY. TAKE EVERY TWO HOURS UNTIL AN IMPROVEMENT OCCURS. REPEAT AS AND WHEN NECESSARY

Peptic ulcers

Peptic ulcers are raw areas that have been eroded by gastric acid and can occur in the stomach or the duodenum. Typically an ulcer causes gnawing upper abdominal pain when the stomach is empty. The pain is normally relieved by eating, drinking or taking an antacid preparation, but occasionally gastric ulcers become more painful after eating. Other symptoms are belching, indigestion or nausea and vomiting, (see pages 90, 92 and 94). *If you suspect an ulcer, you should consult your doctor for medical advice and investigation – urgently if the pain becomes severe, your stools are black or if you are losing weight.*

SYMPTOMS / MEDICINE

❧ A loss of appetite and solid food is vomited. ❧ A constant dull pain. ❧ An aversion to bread and vegetables.	◉ Hydrastis canadensis
❧ Pain in the small area over the stomach. ❧ Vomiting of yellow fluid. ❧ A heavy feeling is felt after eating.	◉ Kali bichromicum
❧ Great hunger, but without any increase in weight. ❧ A need to get up at night to eat. ❧ Regurgitation of sour liquid, which may have a smell of bad eggs.	◉ Psorinum

DOSAGE

USE THE 30C POTENCY. TAKE THREE TIMES A DAY FOR TWO OR THREE DAYS.

Nausea and vomiting

ausea and/or vomiting rarely last for more than 24 hours, but if you have frequent or prolonged episodes of nausea or vomiting, you should consult your doctor so that the cause can be investigated.

However, you need urgent medical advice if, in addition to nausea and/or vomiting, the vomit contains blood or particles that look like coffee grounds, you also have severe abdominal pain, a headache, fever, or have had a recent head injury.

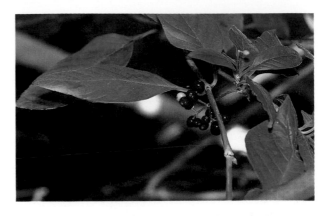

If your nausea is not better after vomiting, Ipecacuanha may bring relief, especially if you are producing copious saliva.

SYMPTOMS / MEDICINE

Symptoms	Medicine
• Indigestion and vomiting after dietary indiscretion. • Nausea that is made worse by drinking. • A white coating on tongue.	◉ Antimonium crudum
• Nausea, vomiting and diarrhea. • Nauseous symptoms brought on by overripe fruit, or food past its best. • A burning discomfort that is relieved by warm drinks.	◉ Arsenicum album
• Nausea from odors, especially eggs and fish. • A distended abdomen.	◉ Colchicum autumnale
• Nausea that is not relieved by being sick. • Strong aversion to food, even to its smell. • Profuse salivation.	◉ Ipecacuanha
• Vomiting occurs 2–3 hours after eating. • Symptoms are brought on by anger, overindulgence in food or alcohol. • Symptoms are relieved by warmth applied to the abdomen or warm drinks.	◉ Nux vomica
• Symptoms are improved by cold drinks, but these are vomited back as soon as they are warmed up in the stomach.	◉ Phosphorus
• Symptoms are brought on by fats, rich food, ice cream and pork. • Lack of thirst. • A desire for open air.	◉ Pulsatilla
• Travel sickness made worse by the thought of food. • Nausea and vomiting accompanied by copious salivation. • A need to lie down.	◉ Cocculus indicus
• Nausea on seeing or smelling food. • Nausea aggravated by cigarette smoke. • Nausea before eating in the morning or after a meal.	◉ Sepia
• Copious vomiting made worse by drinking. • A craving for fruit, cold or acidic drinks. • Nausea gets worse when moving about. • Feels very weak after vomiting.	◉ Veratrum album

DOSAGE

USE THE 30C POTENCY. TAKE THE SELECTED MEDICINE THREE TIMES A DAY FOR TWO OR THREE DAYS.

Diarrhea and colitis

*G*astroenteritis is the inflammation of the digestive tract (see page 87) and it is the most frequent cause of diarrhea. Inflammation that is confined to the colon (part of the large intestine) is called colitis and here the diarrhea usually contains blood and mucus and may also be accompanied by abdominal pain and fever. Colitis is a feature of Crohn's disease and ulcerative colitis. *If you have either of these conditions, you should treat them homeopathically only under the supervision of a doctor.*

SYMPTOMS / MEDICINE

Symptoms	Medicine
❧ Diarrhea after exposure to cold, dry winds or as a result of a fright. ❧ Cold drinks may bring on the diarrhea.	Aconitum napellus
❧ Vomiting at the same time as the diarrhea. ❧ Restlessness and anxiety. ❧ Symptoms are worse during the night. ❧ Thirst for small quantities of warm drinks.	Arsenicum album
❧ Painless, watery, offensive yellow stools. ❧ Diarrhea after eating too much fruit.	Chinchona officinalis
❧ Painful, cramping colic relieved by pressure or by bending double. ❧ Thin, spluttery, copious yellow stools immediately after eating.	Colocynthis
❧ Painless, profuse, watery stools containing undigested food. ❧ Illness may be of a nervous origin.	Phosphoricum acidum
❧ Profuse, spluttery, watery, 'pea soup'-like diarrhea. ❧ Diarrhea is worse in the early morning and is often preceded by painful colic. ❧ Stools are extremely offensive. ❧ Diarrhea is followed by weakness.	Podophyllum peltatum
❧ Morning diarrhea is mixed with wind and the stools are lumpy and watery. ❧ A sudden urging with a fear of being incontinent.	Aloe socotrina
❧ Stools contain blood and mucus. ❧ Pain in the rectum after passing stools.	Cantharis
❧ Green, watery stools when the summer weather turns cool. ❧ Diarrhea comes with damp, cold weather. ❧ Diarrhea in the evening.	Dulcamara
❧ Yellowy, watery stools in the morning after breakfast. ❧ Diarrhea from vegetables and after wet weather.	Natrum sulphuricum

DOSAGE

USE THE 12C POTENCY. TAKE EVERY HOUR UNTIL AN IMPROVEMENT IS MAINTAINED.

Hemorrhoids
Piles

Hemorrhoids can occur at any age, but they are a frequent complication of pregnancy. Internal hemorrhoids are varicose veins occurring in the anal canal. Often, they become external and although these are painless, they may develop a clot within themselves which may be painful. An early symptom of hemorrhoids is anal irritation. There may be a feeling of 'something coming down', particularly after a bowel movement, and in half of the cases there is anal bleeding.

Although hemorrhoids are not a serious medical problem, any unexplained rectal or anal pain, or bleeding, requires early medical diagnosis.

SYMPTOMS / MEDICINE

Symptoms	Medicine
❧ A sensation of splinters in the rectum. ❧ Aching in the lower part of the back. ❧ Purple hemorrhoids. ❧ Burning, itching dryness of the anus. ❧ Anal pain for hours after stools are passed. ❧ Severe lower backache.	◉ Aesculus hippocastanum
❧ Hemorrhoids protrude like a bunch of grapes and bleed easily. ❧ Cold-water applications provide relief. ❧ Marked burning in the anus. ❧ A tendency to diarrhea.	◉ Aloe socotrina
❧ Bluish-colored hemorrhoids. ❧ A stretching pain when walking or sitting. ❧ A burning pain when stools are passed, which is worse for heat.	◉ Arsenicum album
❧ Bleeding hemorrhoids. ❧ Anal burning, itching, smarting and stinging occurs when passing stools.	◉ Capsicum annuum
❧ Painful, bleeding hemorrhoids. ❧ Constipation with no urge to have a bowel movement. ❧ Itching around the anus.	◉ Collinsonia canadensis
❧ Hemorrhoids protrude, burn and sting. ❧ Hemorrhoids are worse when sitting.	◉ Graphites
❧ Hemorrhoids bleed profusely. ❧ Burning, soreness and a sensation of fullness. ❧ Anus feels raw. ❧ Backache and an urging to pass stools.	◉ Hamamelis virginiana
❧ A sharp stitching pain shoots up the rectum. ❧ Hemorrhoids protrude when stools are passed and need pushing back.	◉ Ignatia amara
❧ Painful hemorrhoids.	◉ Millefolium
❧ Bluish, hot, painful hemorrhoids·	◉ Muriaticum acidum
❧ Hemorrhoids and anal prolapse.	◉ Podophyllum peltatum
❧ Anal oozing of soft feces. ❧ Itching and burning with redness around the anus. ❧ Early morning diarrhea on waking.	◉ Sulphur

DOSAGE

USE THE 6C POTENCY. TAKE TWICE A DAY UNTIL AN IMPROVEMENT IS MAINTAINED. FOR THROMBOSED, PAINFUL PILES A DOSE MAY BE TAKEN EVERY THREE HOURS UNTIL THERE IS RELIEF.

Irritable bowel syndrome

(IBS)

*I*BS is said to be the most common reason for people seeking the advice of a doctor specializing in the diseases of the digestive tract. More information is given on page 89. See also the sections on Constipation and Diarrhea, pages 91 and 95.

SYMPTOMS / MEDICINE

Symptoms	Medicine
☙ Considerable stomach distension combined with much gas. ☙ Stools are green, like chopped spinach. ☙ Diarrhea comes on immediately after eating or drinking. ☙ Movements are loose and are made much worse by any anxiety or fear. ☙ Anticipation of an ordeal, such as an examination or an interview, may produce the symptoms.	◉ Argentum nitricum
☙ Diarrhea alternates with constipation. ☙ Stools are slimy with much mucus, but also contain hard lumps. ☙ Tongue becomes coated thick and white. ☙ A craving for acids and pickles.	◉ Antimonium crudum
☙ Diarrhea is frothy, painless and yellow. ☙ Symptoms worse at night and after eating. ☙ Very weak and has a good deal of gas. ☙ Frequent burping does not help to ease the symptoms.	◉ Chinchona officinalis
☙ A painful area just below the belly button. ☙ Stools are loose and are like jelly. ☙ Severe colic pains in the abdomen eased by bending double and pressing on the abdomen, or by applying a hot-water bottle	◉ Colocynthis
☙ Abdomen is painful, rumbling and distended. ☙ Sudden diarrhea with a burning anus. ☙ Cramping pain after stools have been passed.	◉ Gambogia
☙ Stools are either lumpy and covered with mucus, or very loose, brown and mixed with undigested food particles. ☙ Stools are very smelly and have a sour odor.	◉ Graphites
☙ Colic pains in both right and left sides of the abdomen. ☙ Painful constriction of the anus after passing stools. ☙ Diarrhea and pain come on after experiencing a shock or a fright.	◉ Ignatia amara
☙ Stabbing abdominal pains, stools are greenish, bloody and slimy, and all the symptoms are worse at night.	◉ Mercurius solubilis
☙ Loose stools, more frequent during the morning, are yellow and watery. ☙ Large amounts of stool are passed. ☙ Tight clothing around the waist causes burning sensations in the colon and abdominal pain, as if bruised.	◉ Natrum sulphuricum
☙ Early morning diarrhea on waking. ☙ Abdomen is very sensitive to pressure and colic tends to occur after drinking.	◉ Sulphur

DOSAGE

USE THE 12C POTENCY. TAKE EVERY HOUR UNTIL THERE IS AN IMPROVEMENT. REPEAT AS AND WHEN NECESSARY.

CHAPTER 7

THE SKIN, JOINTS & MUSCLES

THE SKIN is the largest organ of the body, accounting for a sixth of body weight. In addition to providing a waterproof cover, the skin protects the body against infection and contains nerve endings that warn the body to withdraw from other physical dangers, such as excessive heat. Some protection against the harmful effects of sunlight is provided by melanin, which is made in the skin, causing it to darken. However, some exposure to sunlight is beneficial (see Osteoporosis, pages 52–53).

Except for the palms of the hands and soles of the feet, the skin bears hairs. Each hair grows out of a tiny pit (the follicle), which occasionally becomes infected, causing a boil.

The skin also contains small glands. Some of these produce a greasy substance called sebum, which keeps the skin supple and waterproof, but may sometimes be produced to excess. Seborrhoeic dermatitis and acne occur more frequently if the skin is greasy. If the opening of one of these glands becomes blocked, the sebum accumulates and forms a sebaceous cyst. This cyst is usually painless unless it becomes infected. Surgical removal under local anesthetic may be needed if a cyst grows too large.

Other glands in the skin produce sweat. Sweating is one of the ways in which the body regulates its temperature and removes certain waste products. Regular exercise enhances this process.

The outer layer of the skin is continually being worn away and replaced by division of the underlying cells. Because this is an active process the health of the skin reflects the general health of the body. Recent research has shown that a number of skin conditions can be improved with mineral and vitamin supplementation. Individual advice may be needed, but following the healthy diet guidelines (see page 88) will certainly help to promote a healthy skin.

JOINTS AND MUSCLES

The joints and muscles form what doctors call the locomotor system of the body: without them we could not move about. Your joints will lose their full range of movement and your muscles will waste away if they are not used regularly. If exercise causes any pain you may need some professional advice about the best way to keep mobile.

ARTHRITIS

Apart from injury (see Emergencies, page 134), the most common problems to affect the joints are the pain, swelling and stiffness caused by the various forms of arthritis. Some of these can also cause painful and stiff muscles.

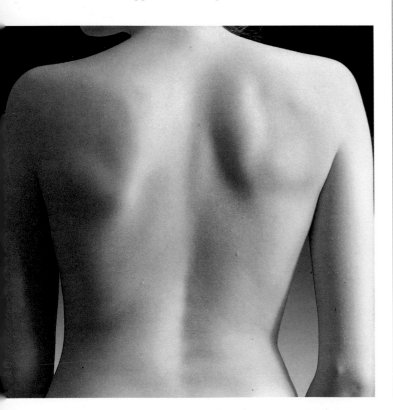

The outer layer of skin is replaced continually as it is worn away. A healthy skin suggests a fit and well-nourished body.

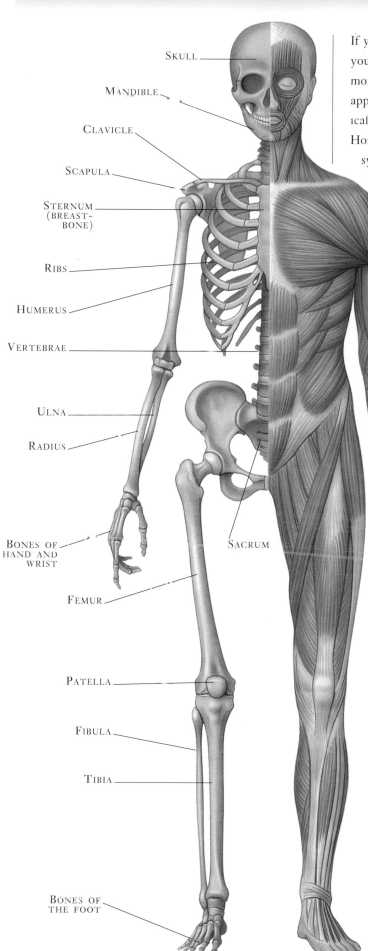

SKULL

MANDIBLE

CLAVICLE

SCAPULA

STERNUM
(BREAST-
BONE)

RIBS

HUMERUS

VERTEBRAE

ULNA

RADIUS

BONES OF
HAND AND
WRIST

SACRUM

FEMUR

PATELLA

FIBULA

TIBIA

BONES OF
THE FOOT

If you develop arthritic symptoms, it is wise to consult your doctor for a formal diagnosis and advice. The more serious forms of arthritis benefit from various approaches, including conventional medication, physical therapy, occupational therapy and acupuncture. Homeopathic treatment is usually constitutional, but symptom medicines are often helpful, particularly for flare-ups of pain that are caused by overuse or changes in the weather.

A number of books advocate dietary changes to combat arthritis. Such changes tend to be regarded as nonsense by many orthodox doctors, but many people do seem to be helped by this approach. It is possible that an individual approach is needed and that different diets will help different people. It is, however, important not to restrict your diet so much that essential nutrients are missing. If in doubt, take professional advice.

FATIGUE

Most people suffer from feeling constantly tired at some stage in life and this feeling is particularly common in early and late pregnancy. At other times you should consult your doctor so that serious causes of exhaustion can be ruled out.

Today there is much publicity about chronic fatigue syndrome (CFS), which is also known as myalgic encephalomyelitis (ME) or post-viral fatigue syndrome (PVFS), and if you feel fatigued, you may worry that you have developed this disabling condition. The most prominent symptoms are usually severe muscle fatigue on or after exertion, and painful muscles and joints. Further information is given on pages 111 and 112. The homeopathic approach is largely constitutional, but symptom medicines can also be useful.

The many muscles in the human body are attached to the bones and enable you to move about and perform everyday tasks. Regular exercise is needed to prevent the muscles becoming stiff and weak.

Acne, boils and pimples

*T*hese types of skin conditions are very common in adolescents, but they can persist into adult life. The eruptions are found mainly on the face, neck and upper chest and back and are caused by inflammation of the small sebaceous glands which open into hair follicles. The glands become blocked and the typical acne rash develops. Infection may occur in some of the spots and these are then likely to feel sore. Boils are inflammatory conditions surrounding a hair follicle. As adolescents frequently have a greasy skin due to bodily hormone changes, it is essential to wash the rash area frequently and thoroughly with soap and hot water to degrease it a little. Eating fewer carbohydrates and high-fat foods, such as potato crisps, french fries and chocolate, and drinking more water are sensible precautions, although not accepted as such by all dermatologists.

SYMPTOMS/MEDICINE

Symptoms	Medicine
❧ Many pimples appear on face, some of which may become small boils. ❧ Frequent indigestion and then tongue becomes coated and white. ❧ Best suited if overweight, thirsty and dislike being touched and looked at.	⊛ Antimonium crudum
❧ Crops of boils may appear anywhere on the body. ❧ Boils are sore at first before the pus forms. ❧ Boils appear which come only partially to a head.	⊛ Arnica montana
❧ Skin becomes very rough and sore with persistent acne. ❧ Complexion is pale and earthy.	⊛ Berberis vulgaris
❧ Recurrent boils and carbuncles.	⊛ Echinacea angustifolia
❧ Throbbing with prickling pains. ❧ Discharge of pus from affected skin.	⊛ Hepar sulphuris calcareum
❧ Bluish-red pustules on the face, neck and shoulders, which leave unsightly scars.	⊛ Kali bromatum
❧ Red, pimply eruptions on the forehead and cheeks which sting when touched. ❧ Generally sensitive to cold.	⊛ Ledum palustre
❧ For girls who suffer from acne and scanty periods.	⊛ Sanguinaria canadensis
❧ Boils occur in crops. ❧ Discharge of pus continues and boils are slow to heal. ❧ Discharge is thin and watery.	⊛ Silicea
❧ Chronic acne with rough, hard skin; spots are itchy, red, sore and frequently become infected. ❧ Water and washing aggravate the spots and skin is aggravated by washing and bathing.	⊛ Sulphur

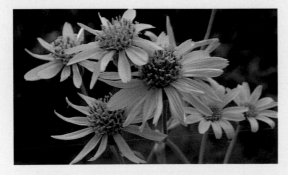

Although Arnica montana is best known for its effective relief of bruising, it can also help to soothe various skin conditions.

DOSAGE

USE THE 6C POTENCY. TAKE TWICE A DAY UNTIL AN IMPROVEMENT OCCURS, THEN STOP. REPEAT THE TREATMENT WITH THE SAME OR ANOTHER MEDICINE, IF INDICATED, AS AND WHEN NECESSARY.

Allergy rashes

*T*hese rashes are known by several different names, but urticaria, nettle rash, poison Ivy and hives are those most frequently used.

A skin eruption, sometimes involving the whole body, may develop quite quickly in response to eating foods such as strawberries and shellfish. The rash that appears on the skin consists of multiple, very itchy pink weals which are smooth and slightly raised. The rash is neither contagious nor infectious *but if the allergy response involves some swelling around the throat or mouth, if the swelling affects the breathing, or if the woman has collapsed, urgent medical attention should be sought immediately.*

SYMPTOMS / MEDICINE

Symptoms	Medicine
☙ Typical hives with intense itching. ☙ Very irritable.	Anacardium orientale
☙ Rash resembles measles.	Antimonium crudum
☙ Feels as if skin is burning and becomes very restless. ☙ Allergy is caused by eating shellfish.	Arsenicum album
☙ Rash, accompanied by diarrhea, occurs after excitement. ☙ Rash develops overnight. ☙ Rash is worse after bathing.	Bovista
☙ Chronic urticaria that is worse from drinking milk. ☙ Feels better in the open air.	Calcarea carbonica
☙ Rash is often accompanied by fever and constipation.	Copaiva officinalis
☙ Chronic allergic rashes which become worse at the start of winter. ☙ Extreme itching on exposure to cold air.	Dulcamara
☙ Urticaria after eating strawberries.	Fragaria vesca
☙ Chronic and recurring urticaria.	Hepar sulphuris calcareum
☙ Nerve rash from stress and anxiety.	Kali bromatum
☙ Rash becomes itchier after exertion.	Natrum muriaticum
☙ Rash appears after eating pork or fruit. ☙ Rash accompanied by diarrhea and chilliness.	Pulsatilla
☙ Rash is red, swollen and intensely irritable. ☙ Rash is better from warmth.	Rhus toxicodendron
☙ Rash after milk or milk products. ☙ Rash is worse in the warmth of the bed.	Sepia
☙ Rash appears after eating shellfish.	Terebinthina
☙ Intense, intolerable itching that is often related to temperature changes. ☙ Itchy swellings of the fingers. ☙ Face becomes blotchy.	Urtica urens

DOSAGE

USE THE 30C POTENCY TAKE EVERY TWO HOURS UNTIL AN IMPROVEMENT OCCURS, THEN STOP. REPEAT AT LONGER TIME INTERVALS, IF NECESSARY.

Eczema

This extremely common condition starts with the affected area of skin showing a greater degree of redness than the surrounding skin. Small, blister-like swellings then develop, and as these rupture they leave crusts or pits which ooze a clear, honey-like fluid. As they heal, they become scaly and very itchy, especially at night in the warmth of the bed. To deal with eczema properly constitutional treatment and dietary advice may be needed.

Eczema is often an indication that other allergies and sensitivities exist in the patient and great care is needed to unravel the totality of the symptoms and provide treatment that is not likely to produce an early aggravation. However, the following symptom treatments will help in alleviating the unpleasantness.

SYMPTOMS/MEDICINE

Symptoms	Medicine
❧ Violently itching eczema. ❧ Feelings of irritability.	◉ Anacardium orientale
❧ Honey yellow-colored crusts. ❧ Skin cracks easily and thick, horny calluses form.	◉ Antimonium crudum
❧ For chronic eczema where skin itches, burns and swells, but in spite of the burning sensation, skin feels better for warm applications. ❧ Feels restless and irritable.	◉ Arsenicum album
❧ Eczema on the scalp, extending to the face. ❧ Crusts are white and very itchy.	◉ Calcarea carbonica
❧ Moist, scabby eruptions on the scalp, face, joints, between the fingers and behind the ears. ❧ Corners of the mouth and eyes become cracked and ooze a gluey, thick, honey-like discharge. ❧ Itching becomes extreme. ❧ Rest of skin may be dry and horny, and the hair is dry and falls out.	◉ Graphites
❧ Moist eczema, especially on the scalp, where it is chronic.	◉ Kali muriaticum
❧ Chronic eczema, which is worse during periods and at the menopause.	◉ Manganum aceticum
❧ There is great itching, which is worse when warm or wrapped up. ❧ Small blisters quickly form scabs and crusts, from which an acrid, thick pus emerges.	◉ Mezereum
❧ Moist eczema without much itching.	◉ Natrum muriaticum
❧ Thick scabs which ooze pus. ❧ Skin is harsh and dry. ❧ Fingertips crack and the hands chap.	◉ Petroleum
❧ Eczema is mainly on head and face, cheeks and ears. ❧ Skin looks dirty, greasy and unwashed.	◉ Psorinum
❧ Eczema with numerous small blisters that itch and tingle. ❧ Worse at night and in damp weather.	◉ Rhus toxicodendron
❧ Skin is rough and coarse with soreness in the folds and violent itching everywhere. ❧ Scalp is dry and hot with intense itching, especially at night. ❧ Scratching causes soreness and burning. ❧ Water and washing make it worse and cause considerable burning and itching.	◉ Sulphur

DOSAGE

USE THE 6C POTENCY. TAKE TWICE A DAY UNTIL AN IMPROVEMENT OCCURS, THEN STOP. REPEAT IF THE SAME SYMPTOMS RETURN.

Itching and skin irritation

Skin irritation can occur without a rash and is occasionally caused by underlying disease, so if it persists consult your doctor. It can be a problem during pregnancy when the skin temperature is slightly raised and a cool bath or shower may give relief. In older women the skin may be itchy because it is rather dry, but using moisturizing creams and lotions can help relieve the problem.

DOSAGE

USE THE 6C POTENCY. TAKE TWICE A DAY UNTIL RELIEF IS MAINTAINED

SYMPTOMS/MEDICINE

Symptoms	Medicine
☙ Skin is dry, itchy and is aggravated by warmth.	◉ Alumina
☙ There is itching of the vagina and vulva.	◉ Caladium seguinum
☙ There is itching all over the body.	◉ Ichthyolum
☙ Itching made worse by undressing.	◉ Rumex crispus

Bunions

This condition, ten times more common in women than in men, is a painful enlargement at the junction of the big toe and the foot. It is probably caused by wearing badly fitting shoes.

SYMPTOMS/MEDICINE

Symptoms	Medicine
☙ A tearing pain in the big toe ☙ May also suffer from gout.	◉ Benzoicum acidum

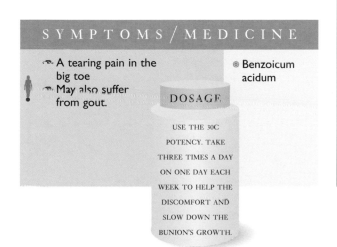

DOSAGE

USE THE 30C POTENCY. TAKE THREE TIMES A DAY ON ONE DAY EACH WEEK TO HELP THE DISCOMFORT AND SLOW DOWN THE BUNION'S GROWTH.

Psoriasis

This is a chronic skin complaint in which red areas covered with scales develop. It is to be found most frequently on the knees and elbows. If the scales are scraped off they produce a shiny, silver sheen which is absolutely typical of this disease. Although these medicines listed below are perfectly satisfactory for immediate treatment, longer term constitutional treatment from a homeopathic doctor will almost certainly be required to improve the condition.

SYMPTOMS/MEDICINE

Symptoms	Medicine
☙ Psoriasis with itching and burning, and it is worse for cold and scratching. ☙ Skin is dry, rough and scaly.	◉ Arsenicum album
☙ Dry, scaly, itchy skin. ☙ Scales peel off easily, leaving a raw surface exposed. ☙ Psoriasis that often occurs in emaciated and elderly women.	◉ Arsenicum iodatum
☙ Pimply, rough, scaly skin. ☙ Eruption appears on scalp and extends to face and neck.	◉ Berberis aquifolium
☙ Skin is unhealthy and any injury suppurates easily. ☙ Psoriasis is better in cold weather.	◉ Borax
☙ There is dry, scaly eruption, especially around eyes and ears.	◉ Chrysarobinum
☙ Rough, thickened skin which may crack. ☙ Fingernails and toenails are also affected. ☙ Much worse in winter.	◉ Petroleum
☙ Yellowish-brown spots appear on the skin. ☙ Itching and rawness.	◉ Sepia
☙ Often helpful for longstanding psoriasis if overweight. ☙ Skin is dry and the hands and feet are cold.	◉ Thyroidinum

DOSAGE

USE THE 12C POTENCY. TAKE TWICE A DAY FOR FOUR WEEKS AND REPEAT AS AND WHEN NECESSARY.

Shingles

This condition is due to infection with the same virus that causes chickenpox. The symptoms are those of a painful eruption, the pain often occurring 2 to 14 days before the rash. The rash appears on one side of the body only, and the initial blotchy red patch, which is rather like a hot-water bottle burn, changes into a collection of small blisters. These eventually crust over to heal in 10–20 days. *Medical attention is needed if the eye and/or the area surrounding it is involved, or if the condition is very painful or extensive.*

SYMPTOMS / MEDICINE

Symptoms	Medicine
• Large blisters with burning and stinging pain. • Cold dressings relieve pain.	◉ Apis mellifica
• Blisters join up together. • Intense burning pain develops which warm dressings relieve. • Restless and feels worse after midnight.	◉ Arsenicum album
• Small, very itchy blisters, which dry quickly producing thick scabs. • Often useful for pain which continues after blisters have healed.	◉ Mezereum
• Severe neuralgic pain in the area affected, which is usually the chest wall. • Clusters of burning, itching blisters which are very tender to the touch and worse with any movement.	◉ Ranunculus bulbosus
• Small blisters with itching and tingling, and surrounding skin appears swollen. • Local warmth helps to ease the pain.	◉ Rhus toxicodendron

Skin ulcers

Skin ulcers usually occur on the legs when the circulation is poor, often as a result of varicose veins (see page 81). Any injury to skin with poor blood supply is likely to become an ulcer, and is normally treated with antiseptic dressings and support bandages. Self-help includes raising the legs above the level of the heart when resting, taking a daily walk, eating a nutritious diet (see page 88) and avoiding standing. If you are applying your own dressings, you can use use Hypericum and Calendula ointment. A number of homeopathic medicines can be used to aid healing, but medical advice is often needed.

SYMPTOMS / MEDICINE

Symptoms	Medicine
• Burning pain that is helped by warmth, and is worse between midnight and 2 am.	◉ Arsenicum album
• Poor circulation, and the leg is cold. • Area feels sore and bruised. • Ulcer is surrounded by a deep bluish-red area.	◉ Hamamelis virginiana
• Edge of the ulcer looks clean cut.	◉ Kali bichromicum
• Skin around the ulcer is bluish-purple. • Ulcer is painful when walking, or being tightly wrapped.	◉ Lachesis mutus
• For when there is infection with foul smelling pus.	◉ Mercurius solubilis **(seek medical advice)**
• Ulcer bleeds easily. • Pain as if a splinter is there.	◉ Nitricum acidum

NITRICUM ACIDUM

Skin infections

Skin infections can occur at any age, and particularly when the skin becomes broken. The more serious skin infections are listed here. Generally, medical help is required if the condition is extensive and spreading, if the regional lymph glands become swollen and painful, if the person becomes toxic (poisoned by the infection) and feverish, or if the face or scalp is involved. Simple skin infections, however, respond well to homeopathic treatment.

Cellulitis is a diffuse inflammation of the subcutaneous tissue of the skin. It appears as redness, swelling, pain and a raised temperature.

Erysipelas is very similar, but is an inflammation caused by a bacteria called the streptococcus, and spreads through the skin and subcutaneous tissues.

Impetigo is an inflammatory, pustular skin disease, usually caused by another bacteria called the staphylococcus. Honey-colored crusts which form on the skin are typical.

You should always consult your doctor for the skin conditions mentioned above.

SYMPTOMS / MEDICINE

Symptoms	Medicine
Bluish-red pustular eruptions.	Antimonium tartaricum
Starts as a light-red discoloration but affected skin soon becomes livid, purple and swollen, and feels bruised and sore. Swelling appears early in the development of the condition.	Apis mellifica
Skin appears bright red and swollen. Skin is smooth, shining and tense. Pain is sharp and throbbing. May also be headache, fever and swollen glands.	Belladonna
Infection starts on nose and spreads to right cheek. Large blisters form which, when they burst, discharge a stinging fluid.	Cantharis
Large yellow blisters. A high temperature. Pain extends from gums to ear.	Euphorbium officinarum
For recurring and chronic cases that involve nose and face. Slightest irritation to skin brings on the condition.	Graphites
Mainly left-sided, the area becomes bright red but soon becomes dark blue/purple. Feels drowsy and weak.	Lachesis mutus
Infection of the skin around the joints. Useful in the early stages of cellulitis.	Manganum aceticum
Infected skin looks dark, red and swollen, and itches and tingles. Small skin blisters appear at the start of the infection. Scalp, face and genitalia are the most common areas involved.	Rhus toxicodendron

DOSAGE

USE THE 30C POTENCY. TAKE EVERY FOUR HOURS UNTIL AN IMPROVEMENT IS MAINTAINED.

Backache and muscle pain

DOSAGE

USE THE 12C POTENCY. TAKEN THREE TIMES A DAY UNTIL THE PAIN STARTS TO SUBSIDE.

*B*ackache is a frequent problem in pregnancy due to the increased weight being carried and the changed stance adopted by pregnant women. However, nearly everyone suffers from backache at some time in their life. It may arise from poor posture or injury, but normally responds well to some form of treatment. Lower back pain or lumbago is a symptom found in many disorders. These range from the common complaint of fibrositis (inflammation of the muscles, usually in the back) to more serious conditions such as a slipped disc where the soft disc between two vertebrae protrudes and presses painfully on the nerve roots. *For continuing or unresponsive back pain, always consult your doctor.*

SYMPTOMS / MEDICINE

Symptoms	Medicine
🦞 A severe, continuous, dull ache in the lower back and hips. 🦞 Back is worse when walking or stooping and may feel that it will give way while walking.	◉ Aesculus hippocastanum
🦞 Muscular pains causing great tiredness. 🦞 Pregnancy vomiting is often associated with the muscle pain.	◉ Aletris farinosa
🦞 Pain as if left side of the abdomen is sprained.	◉ Ammonium muriaticum
🦞 Stiffness and pain in the small of the back. 🦞 Backache is better for complete rest lying on the back to give it support and pressure.	◉ Bryonia
🦞 Suitable for light-haired women who develop back pain and vomiting during pregnancy.	◉ Cocculus indicus
🦞 Severe back pain is experienced which shoots down the buttocks. 🦞 Pain comes on about 3 am, with belief that getting up and moving around will relieve it. 🦞 Back feels weak and stiff. 🦞 Pain arises from feeling cold and lying on the affected side.	◉ Kali carbonicum

Symptoms	Medicine
🦞 Useful for backache after giving birth.	◉ Phosphoricum acidum
🦞 Lower back pain is felt with tiredness.	◉ Pulsatilla
🦞 There is stiffness with or without pain. 🦞 Pain seems to be in the deep back muscles, which feel bruised and hurt on movement. 🦞 Pain feels worse in bed but is better for warmth and improves with some movement.	◉ Rhus toxicodendron

🦞

Care before and after surgery

*H*aving an operation or giving birth can be quite daunting, especially if you are admitted to hospital as an emergency. Some homeopathic medicines can help.

SYMPTOMS / MEDICINE

Symptoms	Medicine
Before operation . . . 🦞 Great fear and anxiety, panic.	◉ Aconitum napellus *30c every 30 minutes as needed*
🦞 Apprehensive, and feels trembly and weak.	◉ Gelsemium sempervirens *30c every 30 minutes as needed*
Before and after operation (including episiotomy or torn perineum) . . . 🦞 To relieve bruising and reduce the risk of infection.	◉ Arnica montana *3 doses the day before the operation, then 30c every two hours for twelve hours after, then four times a day for three days, and then Staphysagria 30c three times a day*
🦞 For bathing wounds after childbirth to keep clean and comfortable.	◉ Hypericum perforatum and Calendula solution.

Hot feet

A burning sensation felt in the feet is a common symptom that may be accompanied by excessive, sometimes offensive, sweating. Modern shoes and socks/tights that are manufactured from synthetic materials, such as plastic or nylon, can make the condition worse. Homeopathic treatment with different medicines is often helpful to reduce the symptoms, but regular washing of the feet and changes of footwear should not be neglected.

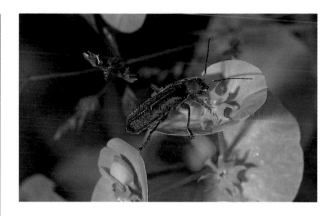

Cantharis, developed from the Spanish fly, can help to cool soles of the feet that are burning.

SYMPTOMS / MEDICINE

Symptoms	Medicine
❧ Offensive foot sweats.	⊛ Ammonium muriaticum
❧ Burning, stinging sensation in feet. ❧ Feet look pinkish and slightly swollen.	⊛ Apis mellifica
❧ Copious and offensive foot sweat. ❧ Cracks may develop, especially on the heels.	⊛ Arundo mauritanica
❧ Cold, clammy, sweaty feet with the toes and soles of feet feeling sore.	⊛ Baryta carbonica
❧ Cold, damp feet accompanied by a sour-smelling sweat. ❧ Cramps in the calves, and even knees feel cold.	⊛ Calcarea carbonica
❧ Soles of the feet are burning, but upper feet are cold and sweaty.	⊛ Cantharis
❧ Feet are sweaty with a tendency to cramps. ❧ Legs are cold from the knees downward.	⊛ Carbo vegetabilis
❧ Cold hands and feet with an acrid foot sweat.	⊛ Iodium
❧ One foot, usually the right, feels hot, while the other feels cold. ❧ Profuse foot sweat, with pain in heels when walking and painful calluses develop on soles of feet.	⊛ Lycopodium clavatum
❧ Smelly foot sweats cause sore toes.	⊛ Nitricum acidum
❧ Feet are hot, eased by putting them outside the bed covers. ❧ May help burning chilblains.	⊛ Pulsatilla
❧ Offensive foot sweats which make the toes sore.	⊛ Sanicula
❧ Profuse foot sweat, often offensive, and may rot socks. ❧ Feet feel hot at night but cold in the day. ❧ Feet feel sore from the instep through to soles.	⊛ Silicea
❧ Burning sensation in the hands and soles of feet. ❧ Feet are hot but are worse at night and better for putting feet outside the bed covers.	⊛ Sulphur

DOSAGE

USE THE 6C POTENCY. TAKE TWICE A DAY UNTIL AN IMPROVEMENT IS MAINTAINED.

Warts

These small, sometimes hard, non-malignant growths occur on the skin, mostly on the hands and fingers, and are caused by a virus. Great care must be taken with hygiene as warts are contagious.

SYMPTOMS / MEDICINE	
ᴈ Skin has a tendency to dryness and may itch in bed.	⊛ Antimonium crudum
ᴈ Large warts appear on fingers, which tend to bleed if damaged. **Consult a doctor.** ᴈ Warts that appear on nose.	⊛ Causticum
ᴈ Large, jagged warts, which may bleed when washed. **Consult a doctor.**	⊛ Nitricum acidum
ᴈ Most frequently used treatment, it can be taken internally or applied as a cream.	⊛ Thuja occidentalis

DOSAGE

USE THE 6C POTENCY. TAKE TWICE A DAY UNTIL AN IMPROVEMENT OCCURS.

ᴈ

Rheumatism and arthritis

Although there are over 250 different joint disorders, homeopathy groups them into the general classification of 'rheumatism' because the picture of these illnesses is very similar. This section therefore contains those medicines most suited to an illness which has joint, muscle or tendon pain, usually stiffness, and sometimes deformity of one or more joints.

The most common form of rheumatism is osteo-arthritis, which is produced by the wear and tear that joints suffer during their use. It is over twice as common as rheumatoid arthritis where the joints become inflamed and painful. *If any doubt exists over the diagnosis or treatment, a doctor should be consulted. Medical help may be needed to treat these conditions.*

SYMPTOMS / MEDICINE	
ᴈ The smaller joints, such as the hands and feet, are those mainly affected. ᴈ Joints ache and swell and the feet are worse for walking.	⊛ Actaea spicata
ᴈ Affected part feels very stiff and sore to the touch. ᴈ Joints swell, making the overlying skin feel stretched and tight. ᴈ Swelling is pale. ᴈ Joints become swollen.	⊛ Apis mellifica
ᴈ Rheumatism that comes about from exposure to damp and cold, with simultaneous muscle strain. ᴈ Affected parts feels sore and bruised.	⊛ Arnica montana
ᴈ Cutting, lightning-like pains run along joints. ᴈ Joints are red, shiny and swollen, and pain radiates through them. ᴈ For rheumatism that is often brought on by getting head and neck wet, or sitting with them exposed to a draught.	⊛ Belladonna
ᴈ Rheumatism in the smaller joints, which develop nodular swellings.	⊛ Benzoicum acidum
ᴈ Acute rheumatism with hot, shiny, dark or pale red joints. ᴈ For pain that is greatly aggravated by movement, but that is relieved by external heat.	⊛ Bryonia
ᴈ Rheumatism that comes on from working in water or damp surroundings. ᴈ Upper back and shoulders are the most affected areas.	⊛ Calcarea carbonica

- Affected joints feel stiff and tight, and lying on them makes them feel sore.
- Pain is worse from cold and is relieved by warmth.
- Restlessness at night, with drawing pains in muscles.
- Ankles are also weak.

⊛ Causticum

- Severe, almost intolerable pain, with compulsion to get up and walk about.

⊛ Chamomilla

- Symptoms are mainly in muscles.

⊛ Cimicifuga racemosa

- Pain is worse in the evenings.
- Affected parts are swollen and dark red.
- Disease moves from joint to joint and typically occurs in debilitated and weak persons.

⊛ Colchicum autumnale

- Rheumatism is worse in changeable weather, especially in damp, cold conditions.

⊛ Dulcamara

- For chronic cases with distorted and knobbly joints.
- Joints are worse from movement and the tendons around them feel tight.

⊛ Guaiacum

- Pain travels upwards, is worse in a warm bed, and affects the smaller joints.
- Any swelling is slight.
- For conditions where nodules form.

⊛ Ledum palustre

- Relief from slow, gentle movement.

⊛ Lycopodium clavatum

- Rheumatism is in the right shoulder.
- Rheumatism is worse in bed or after walking, and better from warmth.

⊛ Magnesia carbonica

- Pain constantly moves from joint to joint.
- Worse in the evening and from warmth but relieved by cold.
- Severe pain that leads to compulsion to move about to try to relieve it.
- Indigestion is also present.

⊛ Pulsatilla

- Rheumatism is worse when there is a weather or temperature change.
- Rheumatism in the chest wall, which feels bruised, although the pain is sharp.

⊛ Ranunculus bulbosus

- Susceptibility to weather change, particularly cold, wintry weather.
- Chronic rheumatism affects the smaller joints, which are worse during rest.
- The parts involved feel weak.

⊛ Rhododendron chrysanthum

- Muscle stiffness and soreness.
- Prominent body projections are tender.
- Pain is worse on first starting to move, worse from sitting and rising from a sitting position.
- Relief from continued movement and warmth.
- Damp weather and damp dwellings aggravate the condition.

⊛ Rhus toxicodendron

- Soreness and lameness that is similar to a tendon sprain.
- Rheumatism of wrists and ankles is present.

⊛ Ruta graveolens

- Acute muscular rheumatism with shifting, sharp, stitching pains and soreness and stiffness in muscles, especially back and neck and right shoulder.

⊛ Sanguinaria canadensis

- Chronic, often familial, rheumatism.
- Pain is worse at night and from uncovering, and is better from warmth.
- Ankles are also weak.

⊛ Silicea

- Acute and chronic rheumatism.
- Inflammation starts in feet, then extends up the body.
- Pain is worse in bed and at night.
- Jerking of the limbs while falling asleep.

⊛ Sulphur

DOSAGE

USE THE 6C POTENCY. TAKE
TWICE A DAY AND STOP WHEN
AN IMPROVEMENT IS
MAINTAINED. THEREAFTER,
PROVIDED IT IS STILL THE
INDICATED MEDICINE, TAKE IF
THERE IS A DETERIORATION.

CHAPTER 8

METABOLIC PROBLEMS

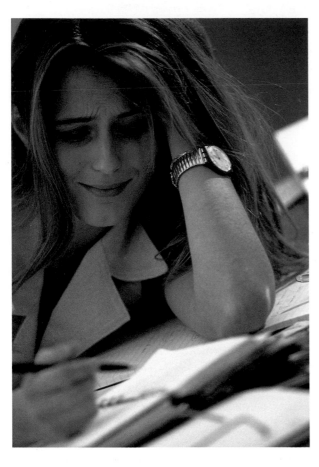

Sufferers of chronic fatigue syndrome often experience a lack of energy which seems to be linked to a metabolic problem.

THE WORD metabolism is used to describe the chemical processes that are continually taking place in the body. These processes include the building up of complex substances, such as proteins, from simpler ones, and the breaking down of complex substances, usually with the release of energy, into simpler ones. The chemical processes of the body take place in every cell and are controlled by proteins, known as enzymes, which often require the help of vitamins and minerals to function effectively.

In health, these processes are balanced. This balance can be lost as a result of inherited abnormalities, disturbances in the secretions of hormones, such as those produced by the thyroid or adrenal glands, or poor nutrition. Metabolic disorders, such as severe diabetes mellitus, can be life threatening and these will usually require conventional treatment. Sometimes no conventional treatment is, as yet, available. Minor metabolic disorders may require no treatment at all.

In chronic fatigue syndrome, the exact metabolic problem has not been identified. A variety of research projects have highlighted possible areas of unbalanced metabolism, and it seems likely that there are several areas where the normal controls are not functioning properly, including those involved in the release of energy within the cells of the body. The response to homeopathy varies greatly, but in some people it seems to be very helpful.

Food intolerance (see page 114) appears to cause disabling fatigue in some people, whether or not their doctors have made a formal diagnosis of chronic fatigue syndrome. Those who are intolerant of alcohol often feel better if they stop drinking. They may find that their energy is further improved if they cut down on the sugar and yeast in their diet. Bread made from dough or sourdough, vinegar and other fermented products, dried fruit and mushrooms are usually the major sources of dietary yeast

Excess weight (see Obesity page 115) is often blamed on 'gland problems'. Occasionally, this is the case, for example when the thyroid gland is not secreting sufficient hormones. For many people the problem is also partly related to the body shape that has been inherited from their parents: the thin types having, apparently, a natural ability to burn up more food without storing fat. Those who store fat easily and attempt to control their weight with long-term low-calorie diets run the risk of eating inadequate amounts of minerals and vitamins, and this can itself be a cause of unbalanced metabolism. This problem is made worse by the modern fashionable emphasis on being slim, which often leads women to try to achieve unrealistic weight goals.

MYALGIC ENCEPHALOMYELITIS (ME)
& other Chronic Fatigue Syndromes (CFSs)

Slow recovery from influenza or some other viral infection is not uncommon, and should not be confused with the more unusual myalgic encephalomyelitis (ME). By convention ME is not normally diagnosed until the symptoms have lasted for more than six months after an infection, and only then after excluding other diseases.

THE NAME IS A DESCRIPTIVE
TERM FOR THE ILLNESS . . .

myalgia	=	muscle pain
enceph-	=	affecting the brain
myel-	=	affecting the nerves
itis	=	inflammation

About 20 per cent of people with ME symptoms show no evidence of infection being the cause. Some of them may be suffering from multiple chemical sensitivities, a controversial condition that is poorly recognized by doctors. The term 'chronic fatigue syndrome' (CFS) will be used here to include all causes.

KEY FEATURES OF CFS (ALWAYS PRESENT)
- Extreme physical and mental fatigue after trivial exertion, and recovering only very slowly.
- Symptoms fluctuate from day to day, or even within one day.

OTHER SYMPTOMS
(NOT ALL PRESENT IN EVERY CASE)
- Muscles: pain and weakness.
- Brain: poor memory, impaired concentration.
- Speech difficulties.
- Emotional variations.
- Sensory changes, for example, oversensitivity to sound or light.
- Severe headaches not helped by painkillers.
- Sleep disturbance.

NERVES REGULATING NORMAL BODILY FUNCTIONS . . .
- Disturbed digestive function, for example, nausea and diarrhea.
- Palpitations, breathlessness and blood-pressure changes.
- Poor temperature control; inappropriate sweating.
- Blurred vision.
- Disturbed bladder function.

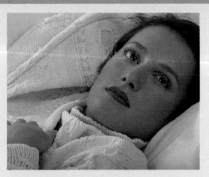

In CFS extreme physical and mental fatigue occurs after just trivial exertion.

MISCELLANEOUS:
- Recurrence or continuing symptoms of original infection.
- Intolerance of alcohol and sometimes foodstuffs.

ADVERSE REACTIONS TO . . .
- Chemicals, including medicines, perfumes, and household cleaning agents.
- Electromagnetic fields, including fluorescent lights and television sets.

SELF-HELP
- Get plenty of physical and mental rest and sleep, particularly in the early stages of the illness.
- Avoid stiffness: move your joints through a full range of movements each day; if you are too weak, ask for help.
- Eat regularly: unprocessed wholefoods, plenty of fruit and vegetables, good quality protein once or twice a day.
- Avoid anything that causes an adverse reaction, including alcohol and caffeine.
- If you have vaginal thrush, ask your doctor to treat you and your partner. The role of thrush/candida in CFS is controversial.
- Read a book about CFS and encourage your family and friends to read one to help them understand your condition.
- Consider complementary medicine, including constitutional homeopathy.
- Try relaxation techniques and/or learn meditation.
- Join a CFS pressure group. The meetings and/or newsletters provide practical help.
- Never give up: over 50 per cent of sufferers get better within five years. Research into CFS is increasing and the cure may be around the corner.

Chronic fatigue syndrome
CFS

It is estimated that there may be well over 300,000 sufferers of this illness in the US alone. Also known as ME and post-viral fatigue syndrome, chronic fatigue syndrome (CFS) often starts with excessive fatigue, muscle pains, headache and sometimes a slightly raised temperature. Extreme weakness of the arms and legs develops. Many other symptoms have also been reported as being related to this little understood condition. The most frequently occurring of these are blurred vision, nausea, anxiety, abnormal periods of weight gain or loss, lack of concentration, confusion, irritability, insomnia, mood swings and noise intolerance. The symptoms may date back to a minor, viral-type illness and can continue for years. There is no single recommended homeopathic medicine of universal benefit in treating the symptoms of CFS and it likely that at some stage constitutional treatment will be necessary. See also Fatigue, page 113, and box on page 111.

SYMPTOMS / MEDICINE

Symptoms	Medicine
❧ Impaired memory, depression, irritability and very easily offended. ❧ General weakness, especially in the legs. ❧ Indigestion and an empty feeling in the stomach, relieved by eating.	◉ Anacardium orientale
❧ Throbbing headache with anxiety and irritability. ❧ Weariness and prostration. ❧ Skin feels cold. ❧ Loss of appetite with a great thirst for water. ❧ Insomnia.	◉ Chininum arsenicosum
❧ Physical and mental exhaustion, with a dislike of meeting people. ❧ Irritable, anxious and very nervous. ❧ Tinnitus (noises in the ear) is often present. ❧ Breath is offensive and mouth is dry. ❧ Stomach feels perpetually empty. ❧ Weakness in back and legs, and the symptoms are worse for exertion.	◉ Kali phosphoricum
❧ Great weakness that is worse in the summer heat. ❧ Mental weakness and difficulties in comprehension. ❧ Sensitivity to noise, and anxiety and restlessness during thunderstorms. ❧ Headache from the least mental exertion. ❧ Very poor digestion. ❧ Legs feel particularly weak in the morning.	◉ Natrum carbonicum
❧ Symptoms start with mental weakness and physical weakness quickly follows. ❧ Apathy and indifference to comprehension difficulties. ❧ Frequent severe headaches that are made worse by noise. ❧ Symptoms are worse after sour food and drink. ❧ Gas and nervous diarrhea. ❧ Frequent urination at night.	◉ Phosphoricum acidum
❧ Weakness with back pain and pins and needles in the legs. ❧ No will-power and a disinclination to work. ❧ Headache is relieved by pressure (firm bandaging). ❧ Limbs feel tired and heavy and feet are cold.	◉ Picricum acidum
❧ Tiredness, depression and impaired memory. ❧ Very sensitive to noise and very chilly. ❧ Ravenous hunger mid-morning. ❧ Lower back pain is worse from sitting. ❧ Feet are in constant motion.	◉ Zincum metallicum

DOSAGE

USE THE 12C POTENCY. TAKE THREE TIMES A DAY UNTIL AN IMPROVEMENT IS MAINTAINED.

Hypoglycemia

hypo-	=	low
glyc-	=	glucose
emia	=	in the blood

If you ask most doctors about hypoglycemia, you are likely to be told that it is rare, except in diabetics who have taken too much insulin. However, many homeopaths recognize a condition that they call 'reactive hypoglycemia' in which the symptoms are similar but less severe. The symptoms often start suddenly, and may appear before breakfast, after missing a meal, two to five hours after eating, or during exercise.

SYMPTOMS OF HYPOGLYCEMIA

- Weakness, faintness, fast heartbeat, cold sweat and dizziness.
- Mental disturbance: anxiety, panic irritability and mood swings.
- Hunger but also nausea.
- Migraines and headaches.
- Waking hungry, raiding kitchen for food at night.

Reactive hypoglycemia requires a constitutional prescription from a homeopathic doctor, but help yourself by:

- Eating wholegrain products in preference to white flour, rice, pasta, etc.
- Eating small meals frequently.
- Cutting out tea, coffee and alcohol.
- Avoiding sugar, chocolate, jam, etc.
- Changing your lifestyle: take plenty of rest, regular exercise and try to reduce stress.

If these measures have not helped after four weeks, check with your doctor.

Brown rice is a wholegrain product, and wholewheat grains are used to make wholewheat bread and brown pasta. By including some of these foods in your diet you can help to relieve hypoglycemia.

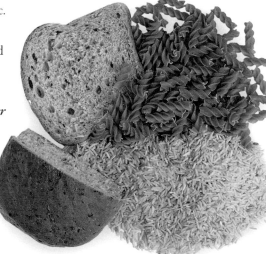

Fatigue

Feeling fatigued after a busy day is perfectly normal but it is not normal to feel exhausted all the time, particularly if this begins to interfere with your work, your family life or social activities. You should spend a few minutes thinking about possible causes for your fatigue because it is often possible to improve matters.

- Are you looking pale? Do you sometimes feel faint? Do you get more short of breath than you used to, or experience palpitations? If you do, you should see your doctor as you may be anemic.
- Are you putting on weight or feeling colder than you used to? Is your hair thinning or your skin dry? Your thyroid may be becoming underactive, so you should see your doctor.
- Are you eating a good diet? See page 88.
- Are you pregnant? Tiredness is very common during early pregnancy but you should tell your doctor or midwife about your symptoms.
- Are you regularly drinking more than three drinks a day of alcohol? Alcohol, even in moderate amounts, can make you depressed: stop for a week and see if you feel better. Also see page 119.
- Do you need a vacation? Overwork and stress can both cause tiredness.
- Do you have one or more of the following symptoms? Poor concentration, indecisiveness, loss of interest in sex, changed appetite, altered sleep pattern or recurrent headaches? If so see Depression, page 126.
- Have you recently had an infection or an operation? You should not expect to be back to normal immediately: take it easy, give yourself time. See also Chronic fatigue syndrome, page 111 and page 112.

Food intolerance

*F*ood intolerance is a term that some doctors use to describe a reaction to a food that cannot be explained by our present knowledge of the immune system. It is, therefore, not strictly a food allergy in the way that, for example, a peanut allergy is. Many doctors dispute the diagnosis altogether. To complicate matters further, the reaction can be any of a wide variety of symptoms including, for example, migraine, joint pain and swelling or irritable bowel syndrome.

Despite the medical controversy, a growing number of people experience symptoms after eating particular foods and get better if they avoid these foods. Unfortunately, the cause or causes of food intolerance are unknown and there are no tests that reliably confirm the diagnosis.

In general, the foods most likely to cause food intolerance are those that are eaten frequently. In Western countries milk and wheat are often the culprits, but corn and soy products are now used widely by food manufacturers and intolerance to these is also increasing. People who suffer from food intolerance often crave the food to which they are intolerant, and this is one reason for weight gain.

The diagnosis of food intolerance is beyond the scope of this book. Unlike true food allergy, which is usually a lifelong condition, food intolerance responds to treatment. This usually consists of avoiding the offending food(s) completely for a time and then testing to see if the reaction still occurs. Most people can reintroduce the food(s) to their diets but it is wise to restrict them to once or twice a week (even with homeopathy, see below).

Homeopathy can be helpful if you suffer from food intolerance. The symptoms will often improve if you take your constitutional medicine (see pages 10–11). In addition, the homeopathically prepared form of the food itself will sometimes 'neutralize' the reaction if you take it before a meal containing the food you react to. Many of the common foods are already available (see table below) and new ones are being prepared, so if the one you want is not on this list check with your homeopathic pharmacy.

Many everyday foods, such as wheat, soy and milk products, have been made into homeopathic medicines.

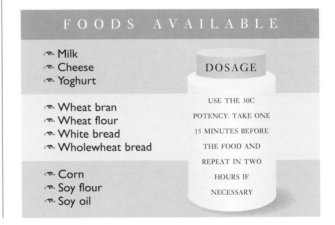

FOODS AVAILABLE

🙟 Milk
🙟 Cheese
🙟 Yoghurt

🙟 Wheat bran
🙟 Wheat flour
🙟 White bread
🙟 Wholewheat bread

🙟 Corn
🙟 Soy flour
🙟 Soy oil

DOSAGE

USE THE 30C POTENCY. TAKE ONE 15 MINUTES BEFORE THE FOOD AND REPEAT IN TWO HOURS IF NECESSARY

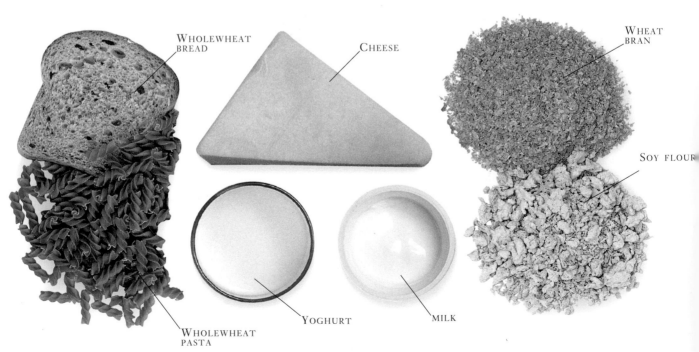

WHOLEWHEAT BREAD

CHEESE

WHEAT BRAN

SOY FLOUR

WHOLEWHEAT PASTA

YOGHURT

MILK

Obesity

For nearly 70 years, calorie counting has been the basis of the majority of slimming diets as it was thought that eating fewer calories than were needed meant that stored fat was burnt up. In the long term, this approach does not work because the body becomes more efficient in the way it ekes out the energy provided by a meagre diet. Once the diet is relaxed, this efficiency persists and the weight goes back on again. Fortunately, a number of doctors are beginning to question this yo-yo approach to slimming and recommend a healthy lifestyle for weight control.

A number of myths persist however. One is that fat people overeat. Some do, but as a group they eat no more than thin people do as a group. Another myth is that you will die sooner if you are fat. Of course it is dangerous to be so fat that you cannot get out of bed, but there is rarely quoted research that suggests that people who are about 30 per cent overweight actually live the longest.

If you are overweight you should take sensible measures to be healthy, including regular exercise (see page 74) and following the advice on healthy eating (see page 88). You should fill up with fruit and vegetables restricting your starchy foods to about four portions a day. You need about three teaspoonfuls of fat a day, preferably in the form of monosaturate or polyunsaturate vegetable oil. Avoid fruit juice as this tends to put your blood sugar up and leads to hypoglycemia (see page 113) and binge eating. In some people, obesity results from food intolerance.

The homeopathic treatment for obesity is constitutional (see pages 10–11). You should consult the *Materia Medica* section which is in the second half of this book (see pages 145–171) to help you select the best medicine to help you.

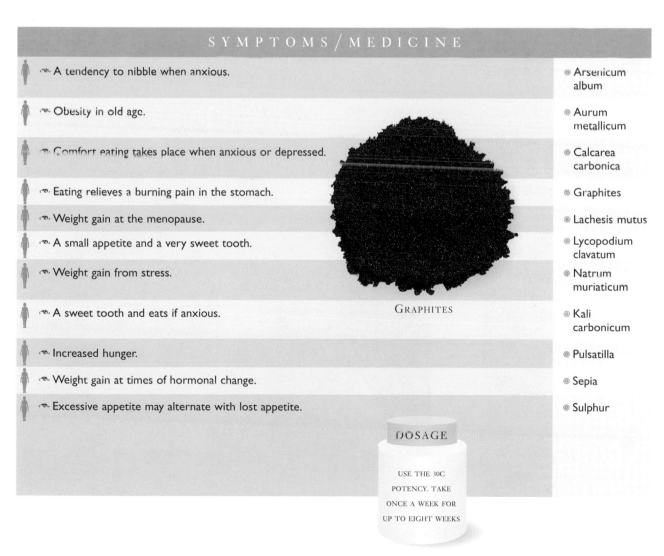

SYMPTOMS / MEDICINE

Symptom	Medicine
A tendency to nibble when anxious.	Arsenicum album
Obesity in old age.	Aurum metallicum
Comfort eating takes place when anxious or depressed.	Calcarea carbonica
Eating relieves a burning pain in the stomach.	Graphites
Weight gain at the menopause.	Lachesis mutus
A small appetite and a very sweet tooth.	Lycopodium clavatum
Weight gain from stress.	Natrum muriaticum
A sweet tooth and eats if anxious.	Kali carbonicum
Increased hunger.	Pulsatilla
Weight gain at times of hormonal change.	Sepia
Excessive appetite may alternate with lost appetite.	Sulphur

GRAPHITES

DOSAGE

USE THE 30C POTENCY. TAKE ONCE A WEEK FOR UP TO EIGHT WEEKS

CHAPTER 9

EMOTIONAL PROBLEMS

THE TERM 'emotional problems' is frequently used to describe a wide range of psychological difficulties. The most common symptoms are depression and anxiety but 'emotional problems' also include many feelings, such as anger, frustration, loss of self-confidence and guilt. You may be more vulnerable to these difficulties if you had an unsatisfactory upbringing but very few, if any, women do not experience emotional stress at some time in their adult life.

Emotional problems are often overwhelming. They are most easily recognized and accepted when they are precipitated by an obvious event, such as a death, job loss or marital breakdown. For many women, asking for help is often far from easy but it is important not to suppress your feelings because this can store up trouble for later.

Some women have the extra difficulty of living through a range of emotional pressures that depend to some extent on their hormone levels. They may experience considerable emotional distress as a result of premenstrual syndrome, painful periods, pregnancy, childbirth or the menopause.

Homeopathy is particularly well suited to relieving emotional problems. Symptom medicines will often be helpful for the minor ups and downs of life, and constitutional treatment has, of course, a much wider range of action. The more serious emotional problems should only be treated with homeopathy if there is medical supervision. If you are unfortunate enough to suffer from a

CALCAREA
PHOSPHORICA

psychiatric illness, you may still suffer from the same emotional problems as everyone else, and you may find that homeopathy will help you through the problems discussed in this chapter. Homeopathic medicines can be taken along with other medication, but discuss this with your doctor.

DEPRESSION

Depression is a normal response to a sad event, or to a series of mishaps. If you experience the symptoms of mild depression, such as feeling low, tired, irritable or frustrated, you may well find a homeopathic medicine that helps. More serious depression is indicated by changes in appetite, loss of sexual desire, sleep disturbance and thoughts of suicide. It is often helped by constitutional prescribing, but this requires medical supervision.

ANXIETY

Anxiety is a perfectly normal emotion and can range from a feeling of mild unease to that of intense fear. Because anxiety is an unpleasant feeling it can have the beneficial effect of stimulating you to avoid or remove the cause. It is only when anxiety disrupts your everyday activities that it becomes a problem. Then it can take over your thoughts and will often lead to an irrational feeling that something bad will happen. Anxiety can cause physical symptoms including palpitations, chest pains, muscle tension, digestive upsets, frequency in urination, sweating, blushing and fatigue. It is important to discuss your symptoms fully with your doctor because so many of these symptoms can also be caused by physical illness. (See also page 124.)

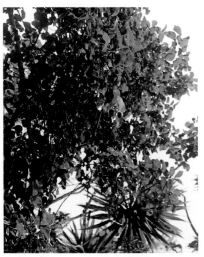

Once used by conventional doctors to improve appetite, Nux vomica has become an important homeopathic medicine.

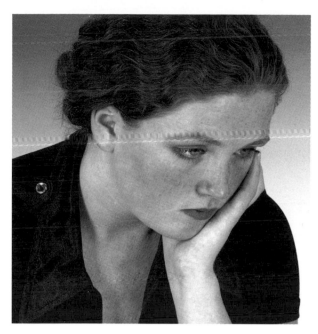

Anxiety is an unpleasant feeling, but it can have the beneficial effect of stimulating you to avoid or remove the cause.

PANIC ATTACKS

A panic attack is a brief period of intense anxiety in which you feel that you will die or lose your reason. At first these attacks are unpredictable but, eventually, they become associated with certain places, such as a crowded bus. The physical symptoms are those of anxiety and may in particular include overbreathing (hyperventilation). This can often be helped by breathing in and out of a paper bag for a few minutes.

POST-TRAUMATIC STRESS DISORDER

This type of anxiety occurs either immediately after a frightening event, or some months later. Such events include natural disasters, serious accidents, rape and other violent attacks. The symptoms include feelings of guilt, dreams or recurring memories of the event and a sense of isolation. Homeopathy is often beneficial for panic attacks and post-traumatic stress because the idea of never having been the same, or felt normal, since an event can be a strong indication for a certain medicine. Some of these are discussed in this chapter.

PHOBIA

The word phobia means 'fear', but it is usually used to describe an ongoing and irrational fear of something, which may be an object, an animal or a situation. It is a very common experience: most people are afraid of spiders or snakes, for example, and this characteristic can be very useful in determining which constitutional medicine to prescribe. A phobia only becomes a problem when it interferes with normal life, and then it usually needs professional treatment. (See page 129.)

EATING DISORDERS

The relationship between women and food is very complex. Eating is no longer a matter of survival but has become a social event, and most meals are prepared by women. A woman is expected to be a good cook and also to nurture her children by giving them adequate and interesting food as part of being a 'good mother'. The provision and preparation of food has thus become closely associated with a woman's feelings about her role in life and how well she is doing.

On a personal level, women can become obsessed by food. Appetite is normally controlled by feelings of hunger before a meal, and satisfaction afterwards. It is, therefore, not surprising that women often turn to food when they are feeling depressed or in need of comfort.

❧ *Obesity* is not just the result of overeating: it can result from too much 'slimming'. It has been recognized that, in some women, severe calorie restriction stimulates the body into becoming very efficient so a return to a normal calorie intake after a period of dieting is accompanied by weight gain. A further complication, in Western countries at least, is the social pressure to be thinner than is sensible or healthy. Fortunately, the growing awareness of healthy eating is creating a more balanced approach to 'slimming' with realistic goals for weight, and diets that contain adequate amounts of minerals and vitamins.

❧ *Anorexia nervosa and bulimia nervosa* are eating disorders that appear to be becoming increasingly common. In anorexia there is an overwhelming fear of being fat, so food is avoided and there is a serious, sometimes fatal, loss of weight. In bulimia, bouts of overeating are followed by self-induced vomiting, which is usually done in secret. Although bulimics are often of normal, or near-normal, weight, they can endanger their lives by becoming dehydrated, and the loss of potassium from their bodies can cause weakness. The diagnosis is sometimes made by dentists since the repeated vomiting of the acidic stomach contents may damage the teeth. Homeopathic medicines can be useful for eating disorders, but anorexia and bulimia should be treated only under medical supervision. (See also page 120 and page 122.)

DRUG DEPENDENCE

A drug is a chemical substance that is known to alter the way the body functions and/or to change the course of a disease. Such substances are present in tea, coffee, alcohol and cigarettes, and are often used to excess by people under stress. Recreational drugs are being increasingly used for relaxation, particularly by young people (see page 121).

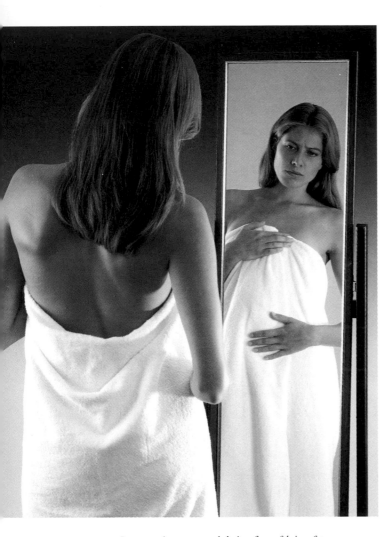

In anorexia, an overwhelming fear of being fat can cause a distorted impression of the body image.

DON'T DEPEND ON STIMULANTS

Many people looking for ways to ease the stresses of life turn to caffeine, alcohol and sugar. Although these may be beneficial in small amounts, in greater quantities they may damage your health.

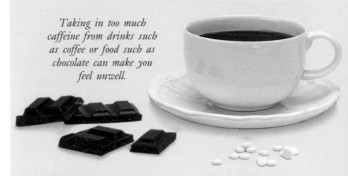

Taking in too much caffeine from drinks such as coffee or food such as chocolate can make you feel unwell.

CAFFEINE
Found in coffee, tea, cola, chocolate, some painkilling drugs.

BENEFITS
- Reduces fatigue, aids concentration.
- May relieve asthma.
- Enhances simple painkillers.
- Minerals such as manganese and fluoride are also present in tea.

ADVERSE EFFECTS
- Can cause anxiety, panic attacks, nervousness depression, irritability and insomnia.
- Tremor and palpitations can be side effects.
- Can bring on indigestion, diarrhea and also raised cholesterol.
- Iron and zinc deficiency if tea or coffee is taken with meals.
- Can bring on migraines or withdrawal headaches.
- Restless legs particularly at night can be a side effect.
- Can cause painful or lumpy breasts
- Can make a baby unsettled if you are breast-feeding.

SELF-HELP . . .if you think less caffeine would help you, withdraw gradually to avoid headaches.

ALCOHOL

Virtually every organ in the body can be damaged, often seriously, if you regularly have more than three drinks a day. If you drink more than this you should cut down as a priority. One drink of alcohol is a glass of table wine, a small glass of sherry, 12 ounces of beer or an ounce of hard liquor.

BENEFITS

🕸 The chances of osteoporosis, heart disease and strokes may all be reduced by having 1 to 2 drinks a day, but drinking more increases the risk. In heart disease the benefit is greater with wine than with beer or hard liquor.

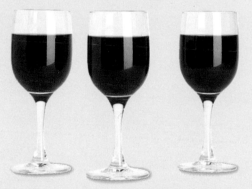

If you regularly have more than three drinks of alcohol a day you should cut down as soon as you can.

ADVERSE EFFECTS OF MODERATE DRINKING

🕸 Obesity: calories from alcohol convert easily to fat.

🕸 Nutritional deficits: your body requires more vitamins and minerals.

🕸 Breast cancer and high blood pressure: the risks are increased by drinking more than one alcoholic drink a day.

🕸 Panic attacks can be triggered by alcohol in susceptible individuals.

🕸 Hot flushes occur more frequently after alcohol.

TIPS FOR MODERATE DRINKING

🕸 Have two alcohol-free days a week.

🕸 Quench your thirst first with a non-alcoholic drink.

🕸 Dilute your drinks by using a mixer, and drink slowly.

🕸 Say no to that last drink, or make it a soft drink.

🕸 Record your drinks by keeping a diary, eat a good diet, don't skip meals, and never replace a meal with alcohol on its own.

🕸 Replace evenings at the pub with a hobby, sport etc.

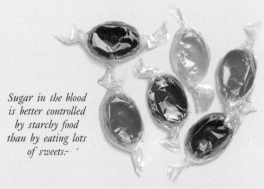

Sugar in the blood is better controlled by starchy food than by eating lots of sweets.

SUGAR

Although sugar has the reputation of giving you a lift, its action is sedative, possibly by increasing serotonin, which acts as a sedative in the brain. Sugar is best taken indirectly as starch, which the body then breaks down into sugar.

BENEFITS

🕸 Relief of premenstrual syndrome: regular meals or snacks of starchy foods benefit many women. Do not take fat and protein at the same time.

ADVERSE EFFECTS

🕸 These include poor control of blood sugar and obesity, but they are largely overcome by eating starchy foods rather than sugar.

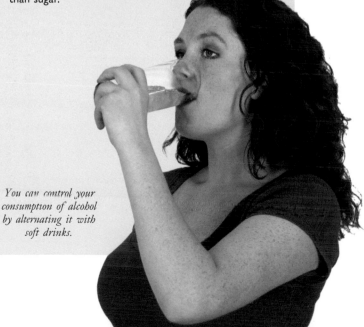

You can control your consumption of alcohol by alternating it with soft drinks.

Anorexia nervosa

*T*his is a serious disorder, much more complicated than a simple loss of appetite, and indicates a psychological aversion to food. The disorder usually, but not always, occurs in adolescent girls who fear becoming fat and develop a distorted impression of their own body image. In fact, at the start of the illness, sufferers are often perfectly normal in size and weight. Anorexia nervosa is characterized by rapid weight loss and inevitably leads to body weakness and general apathy. During the illness the menstrual periods often become quite irregular and may even stop completely.

It is vital that medical advice is sought as early as possible following the onset of the illness. Some people suffering from anorexia nervosa need to be admitted to hospital for treatment.

SYMPTOMS / MEDICINE

Symptoms	Medicine
❧ Complete and almost total loathing of food and drink. ❧ Tendency to be overweight at the start of the illness. ❧ Tendency to be sentimental and dislikes being touched. ❧ May feel peevish, sad and weepy.	⊛ Antimonium crudum
❧ Can help nervous and anxious people, who are excitable or melancholic and oversensitive to noise. ❧ Nausea and constantly yawning. ❧ A desire for alcohol.	⊛ Asarum europaeum
❧ Following a total loss of appetite, lips and tongue become very dry and constipation develops with hard, dry stools. ❧ Cannot bear any disturbance or movement and wants to be left alone, becoming irritable, angry and nervous if disturbed.	⊛ Bryonia
❧ Affects tall, usually slim women, the illness often follows grief or an unfortunate love affair. ❧ Complains of colicky abdominal pains when trying to eat.	⊛ Calcarea phosphorica
❧ Anorexia often follows a debilitating illness. ❧ May appear pale and greyish and have a poor memory and slow thought processes. ❧ Stomach feels full after the smallest amount of food or drink and can become very distended with wind.	⊛ Carbo vegetabilis
❧ Total aversion to the sight or smell of food, and bright lights and noise become unbearable. ❧ The illness often comes on after grief.	⊛ Colchicum autumnale
❧ Sulky and despises everything. ❧ Continual nausea which is not made any better by vomiting. ❧ Despite vomiting, tongue is clean. ❧ Profuse salivation may be present.	⊛ Ipecacuanha
❧ Any slight appetite disappears on eating the first mouthful of food, especially cold food. ❧ Tendency to become very apprehensive, weepy and cannot bear to be contradicted. ❧ Symptoms are worse between 4 and 8 pm. ❧ The illness may follow a fright or anger.	⊛ Lycopodium clavatum
❧ Anorexia begins after suffering grief, fear or extreme anger. ❧ Intolerant of any help or consolation. ❧ Terrible headaches, which come on during the day and recede in the early evening. ❧ Tongue feels numb and tingles. ❧ Acne and greasy skin.	⊛ Natrum muriaticum
❧ Food is vomited as soon as it reaches stomach. ❧ Suitable for tall, slim, sensitive, artistic types who are oversensitive to light, noise, smells and touch. ❧ Restless and fidgety. ❧ Great weakness and loss of strength.	⊛ Phosphorus

- ✿ Fear that food is poisonous and becomes very restless, anxious and apprehensive, especially at night.
- ✿ Dizziness when walking or standing.

◉ Rhus toxicodendron

- ✿ Nausea from the smell of food cooking.
- ✿ A tendency to faint very easily.
- ✿ Very sad and weepy feelings, with indifference to family and friends, but there is a dread of being alone.
- ✿ A continual empty feeling in the stomach which is not relieved by eating.

◉ Sepia

- ✿ Complete appetite loss with sour burping and great acidity in the stomach.
- ✿ Skin is unhealthy with acne and itching, which gets worse when scratched or washed.
- ✿ Selfish, irritable and argumentative.
- ✿ A sensation of weakness that is worst mid-morning.
- ✿ Abdomen is very sensitive to pressure.

◉ Sulphur

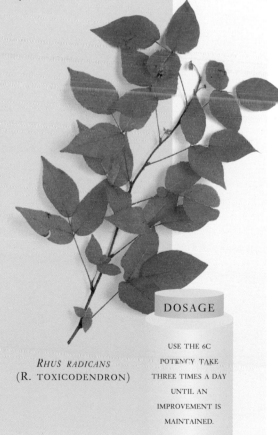

RHUS RADICANS
(R. TOXICODENDRON)

DOSAGE

USE THE 6C POTENCY TAKE THREE TIMES A DAY UNTIL AN IMPROVEMENT IS MAINTAINED.

Drug abuse

Drug abuse is an increasing problem and applies to all drugs whether illegal 'designer drugs' taken to produce a 'buzz' in a social situation or prescribed drugs taken, for example, to help someone to sleep or to counteract the effects of extreme stress. Unfortunately, many of these drugs can have serious side effects and can also become so habit forming that a higher and higher dose has to be taken to produce the same effect. Some of the drugs are addictive and dangerous and may even lead to death in a susceptible woman. The physical and moral degradation that addicts, for this is what they become, sink to is heartbreaking to their friends and family. *Skilled medical attention is vital as soon as the problem becomes known.* The concurrent use of the following homeopathic medicines may also assist in the treatment of these very unfortunate people.

DOSAGE

USE THE 12C POTENCY. TAKE THREE TIMES A DAY UNTIL AN IMPROVEMENT IS OBVIOUS. RESTART TREATMENT IF AND WHEN NECESSARY.

SYMPTOMS / MEDICINE

- ✿ Easily addicted to stimulants.
- ✿ Peevish, sleepless, want to be left alone.

◉ Capsicum annuum

- ✿ Apathetic.
- ✿ Sense of smell is very acute.
- ✿ A desire for stimulants and tobacco.

◉ Carbolicum acidum

- ✿ Uncontrollable laughter.
- ✿ Aversion to all food but there is a craving for black coffee.
- ✿ Hysteria is apparent.

◉ Moschus

- ✿ This is the homeopathic medicine most frequently indicated for drug abuse.
- ✿ Irritable and can't stand bright lights or noise.
- ✿ Fault-finding.
- ✿ Frequent stomach upsets.

◉ Nux vomica

- ✿ Very sensitive.
- ✿ A preoccupation with sexual problems.
- ✿ A craving for tobacco as well as other drugs.

◉ Staphysagria

Bulimia nervosa
Binge-eating

*I*n this condition the desire to eat is constant. Large quantities of food are devoured, often with no regard for what it is, and the whole process of eating becomes morbid. Eating binges are frequently followed by self-induced vomiting or taking laxatives so that no weight gain is noticed. Unfortunately, the loss of body fluids that occurs may also upset the body chemistry.

It is as serious a condition as anorexia nervosa and medical advice should be sought as the cause is frequently a deep-rooted psychological problem. See also page 120.

SYMPTOMS / MEDICINE

Symptoms	Medicine
❧ A yearning for indigestible things like chalk, dry foods and coffee grounds, but potatoes are often disagreeable. ❧ Dark, slimly built women, who are usually cheerful, but who may have a tendency to be anxious about their health. ❧ All bodily functions are sluggish.	◉ Alumina
❧ May be oversensitive, weak and pale and vomit immediately after eating and frequently during the night as well, usually after midnight. ❧ An aversion to sour foods and an intolerance of eggs. ❧ The slightest noise is unbearable.	◉ Ferrum metallicum
❧ Despite a ravenous hunger and eating habits, there is a failure to gain weight. ❧ Become worried and anxious if they don't eat. ❧ May fear people and social events, and want to give up on life.	◉ Iodium
❧ The more that is eaten, the more is wanted, but feels full after a few mouthfuls. ❧ Excessive gas. ❧ Intellectually keen but physically weak, with the worst time being from 4 to 8 pm. ❧ Peevish and irritable and easily angered.	◉ Lycopodium clavatum
❧ A craving for acidic things and lemonade, with a tremendous thirst. ❧ Very irritable with a nervous temperament and may be thin and lack energy. ❧ Skin feels cold yet cannot bear being covered.	◉ Secale cornutum
❧ Eats very quickly, literally pushing food into mouth. ❧ Symptoms are worse around midday, when feels very weak and debilitated. ❧ Incessant movement of legs and feet. ❧ Generally feels worse after drinking wine.	◉ Zincum metallicum

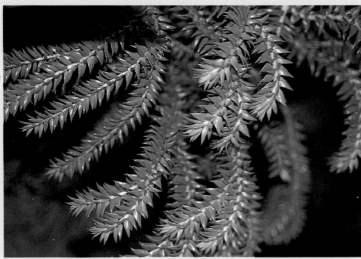

Feelings of great hunger that change to being uncomfortably full after a few mouthfuls of food, can be relieved by taking Lycopodium.

DOSAGE

USE THE 12C POTENCY. TAKE THREE TIMES A DAY UNTIL THERE IS AN IMPROVEMENT, THEREAFTER AT THE FIRST INDICATION OF A RELAPSE.

Alcohol abuse

*M*any women find the relaxing efects of an alcoholic drink a great pleasure at the end of a hard day's work, and provided it is no more than this, overindulgence is unlikely. However, it is very easy to extend the one drink to two and then several, and a pattern can develop of needing a drink to relax. Alcohol abuse has then begun. Sometimes a well developed hangover may act as a deterrent to future excess in some women, but this does not apply to all, so some of the following homeopathic medicines may prove useful in relieving the symptoms.

If the alcohol abuse becomes serious, medical attention should always be sought as soon as possible.

SYMPTOMS / MEDICINE

Symptoms	Medicine
🞬 Irritable and peevish, or sad and weepy, cannot bear to be touched. 🞬 A severe headache and an upset stomach after drinking too much alcohol, especially wine.	◉ Antimonium crudum
🞬 Stomach feels as if it is on fire, which leads to anxiety, irritability and restlessness. 🞬 Indigestion, which is commonly associated with diarrhea.	◉ Arsenicum album
🞬 A strong craving for alcoholic drinks. 🞬 Oversensitivity to all external stimuli. 🞬 Feels better for washing in cold water.	◉ Asarum europaeum
🞬 Nausea and vomiting following overindulgence; the vomit is green and acidic. 🞬 Great despondency and apathy.	◉ Carduus marianus
🞬 A craving for alcohol after loss of sleep while caring for a loved one.	◉ Cocculus indicus
🞬 A liking for effervescent alcoholic drinks. 🞬 Smell of food causes nausea. 🞬 A headache develops which is worse in the late afternoon and evening.	◉ Colchium autumnale
🞬 Sad and quarrelsome, averse to contradiction and no inclination to work. 🞬 Eyes hurt in bright light and there are feelings of dizziness on lying down or turning in bed.	◉ Conium maculatum
🞬 Sedentary, thin, irritable, impatient, angry and spiteful 🞬 Worries about own health and oversensitive to noise, smells, light and music. 🞬 Constant nausea with a feeling that a good vomit would lead to feeling better. 🞬 Indigestion soon after eating, making abdomen very sensitive to pressure.	◉ Nux vomica
🞬 A hangover with aches and pains all over the body but especially in the chest. 🞬 Eyes seem to have a mist over them. 🞬 Skin burns and itches.	◉ Ranunculus bulbosus
🞬 A craving for alcoholic drinks, but these produce severe, right-sided headaches, with burping and vomiting, the taste of which is sour. 🞬 An aversion to the smell of coffee.	◉ Sulphuricum acidum

DOSAGE

USE THE 30C POTENCY. TAKE EVERY TWO HOURS UNTIL RELIEF IS FELT.

Anxiety

Anxiety is normal, but it can become a problem when it disrupts your everyday activities. If you find yourself worrying all the time, particularly if your sleep is disturbed, you may find that going regularly to relaxation classes or taking up yoga helps you to control your thoughts. Vigorous exercise can also be helpful as it releases tension and stimulates the release of endorphins – the body's 'happy' hormones (see also Fright and Panic, page 127 and page 128).

SYMPTOMS / MEDICINE

Symptoms	Medicine
• Great anxiety and restlessness. • A fear that something will happen. • Worse around midnight.	Arsenicum album
• Apprehension and dread of the future. • Despair of getting better. • Irritable feelings and a desire to be left alone.	Bryonia
• Feelings of apprehension towards the evening, and fear of loss of reason.	Calcarea carbonica
• Fear that others will observe this confusion of mind. • Deeply affected by sad stories. • Fear that something will happen. • Intensely sympathetic to the suffering of others.	Causticum
• Anxiety about undertaking new things, health, conflict and career, an aversion to company yet a need to have someone in the next room. • Stage fright.	Lycopodium clavatum
• Tremendous anxiety about health and a dread of serious disease. • Irritable and peevish, especially early in the morning.	Nitricum acidum
• Many fears especially about thunderstorms, something bad happening, or the dark. • Easily startled. • A need for company, and sympathetic to others.	Phosphorus
• Fearful of being abandoned, yet needing reassurance. • Prone to weeping. • A fear of heights, of being shut in, of the dark and of robbers.	Pulsatilla
• Pessimistic, restless anxiety about the future. • A fear of poverty, cancer or failure. • Great anxiety at night.	Psorinum
• Restlessness – both mental and physical. • Anxiety about the children. • Superstitious feelings and a fear of accidentally killing someone.	Rhus toxicodendron
• Anxiety about health, the future, accidents or disease in the family. • Low self-confidence.	Sulphur

DOSAGE

USE THE 30C POTENCY. TAKE EVERY TWO HOURS FOR UP TO SIX DOSES UNTIL THE ANXIETY IS RELIEVED.

Concentration problems

*A*s people get older, the ability to focus attention on any particular problem tends to become more difficult. The mind feels incapable of sustained effort and the capacity to concentrate on difficult problems becomes reduced. Inability to concentrate is a natural symptom of the ageing process, and in itself should not cause undue concern.

SYMPTOMS/MEDICINE

Symptoms	Medicine
❧ Forgetful, easily irritated and depressed.	◉ Ichthyolum
❧ Difficulties in concentrating the thoughts.	◉ Iridium metallicum
❧ Finds it difficult to sustain any length of conversation.	◉ Medorrhinum
❧ Lacks the power to concentrate for long. ❧ Coordination is poor.	◉ Onosmodium virginianum
❧ Lack of self-control and concentration ability.	◉ Opium (prescription required in USA)
❧ Impossible to concentrate which as a result leads to feelings of despondency. ❧ A great desire to be with other people.	◉ Skatolum
❧ Tiredness and an inability to think properly.	◉ Terebinthina

DOSAGE

USE THE 6C POTENCY. TAKE THREE TIMES A DAY FOR FIVE DAYS, THEN REPEAT AS AND WHEN NECESSARY.

Lack of Confidence

A lack of self-confidence can turn a very capable and competent individual into a negative person who doubts, without cause, her ability to perform normal day-to-day activities. At worst she will not even attempt out-of-the-ordinary tasks.

SYMPTOMS/MEDICINE

Symptoms	Medicine
❧ An aversion to work and an irresistible desire to swear and curse. ❧ Lacking confidence in self as well as in others.	◉ Anacardium orientale
❧ A dread of ordeals and feelings of failure. ❧ Impulsive and hurried, with a feeling that time is passing very slowly.	◉ Argentum nitricum
❧ A feeling that no-one has confidence in her. ❧ There are feelings of worthlessness.	◉ Aurum metallicum
❧ A loss of self-confidence for a specific task.	◉ Baryta carbonica
❧ Absent-mindedness, irritability and irresoluteness, and may also become quite fearful.	◉ Calcarea silicata
❧ Lack of courage, and diarrhea in anticipation of an event. ❧ A dread of appearing in public, and there is a fear of losing self-control.	◉ Gelsemium sempervirens
❧ Loss of self-confidence leads to melancholia and fear of being left alone.	◉ Lycopodium clavatum

DOSAGE

USE THE 30C POTENCY. TAKE THREE TIMES A DAY FOR FOUR DAYS, THEN USE WHEN NECESSARY, TAKING THREE DOSES DAILY UNTIL AN IMPROVEMENT IS MAINTAINED.

Clinical depression

*I*t is not abnormal, at times, to feel depressed about some aspect of life. This minor dissatisfaction lasts for a short time, is not severe and only slightly affects our relationships with other people. Clinical depression is, however, a very serious illness which needs skilled professional help. It can last for several weeks or months. The symptoms are sometimes slow to be noticed and may at first show as a lack of self-confidence, increasing apathy, and a lack of emotion.

The symptoms of clinical depression are worse in the morning after waking and tend to lighten as the day progresses. Sleep problems, and especially waking in the early hours, are common and this is coupled with apathy, loss of concentration, lack of sex drive, loss of appetite (sometimes the reverse occurs), constipation and maybe symptoms of illness in other parts of the body. These are psychosomatic (imagined) symptoms and do not indicate actual illness, but they are very real to the sufferer and may be so frightening that they lead to attempts at suicide.

Depression can seriously disrupt life for the patients and affect their relationships with other people, usually their immediate family. The homeopathic medicines suggested below should be used only in simple cases of depression, and the patient should be carefully observed for any deterioration.

Skilled medical attention is vital for all but the mildest cases although homeopathic medicines may be used at the same time. See also Anxiety, page 124.

SYMPTOMS/MEDICINE

Symptoms	Medicine
• Feelings are much worse after listening to music. • A fear of going out, of crowds, of crossing the road and of death. In fact, life becomes intolerable because of these fears. • Anxious, restless and hurried.	◉ Aconitum napellus
• Extremely miserable, imagining all sorts of illnesses. • A great tendency and desire to swear. • Impaired memory. • Very easily offended. • Almost total loss of confidence.	◉ Anacardium orientale
• Mentally very restless with great anguish and fear, especially of dying. • May feel no treatment can help. • The worst time is midnight to 3 am.	◉ Arsenicum album
• Disgusted with life and may think of committing suicide. • Oversensitivity to noise. • Intolerance of the slightest contradiction. • Depressed from grief and disappointed love.	◉ Aurum metallicum
• Sad and hopeless, the slightest thing causes tears. • Can help women with dark hair and eyes who are delicate, sensitive people. • Depression follows grief, loss of sleep and sudden emotional situations.	◉ Causticum
• Despairing, may also feel melancholic and full of anguish. • Menstruation may cease.	◉ Helleborus niger
• Nervous and sensitive, apt to be easily excited and easily offended. • Feelings of mental exhaustion. • Full of contradictions such as laughing at sad news. • Tearful with very rapidly changing moods.	◉ Ignatia amara
• The worst time is immediately after sleep. • No desire for company. • Depressed, but also excitable, engaging in non-stop talking. • Averse to being touched, or wearing tight clothes.	◉ Lachesis mutus

- Extreme depression.
- Convinced is suffering from an incurable disease.
- Timid and tearful, also indifferent to what is being done for them.
- May feel hurried and that life is aimless.

⊛ Lilium tigrinum

- Extreme sadness in the morning on waking.
- Loss of self-confidence.
- A fear of being alone.
- Extreme apprehension.
- The worst time is 4–8 pm.
- Physical weakness.

⊛ Lycopodium clavatum

- Great sadness.
- Depression occurs because of a chronic illness.
- Any consolation makes things worse.
- Feelings of irritability and cries easily.
- Dreams of being robbed.

⊛ Natrum muriaticum

- Sad feelings occur after listening to lively music.
- Gloomy and irritable, there is no wish to speak or listen to others.
- Fed up with life.
- The illness often follows a previous head injury.

⊛ Natrum sulphuricum

- Sad and cries easily.
- Changeable, and contradictory moods.
- Symptoms are better outside.

⊛ Pulsatilla

- Mentally listless and depressed, as well as physically restless.
- Becomes frightened during the night
- Frequent suicidal thoughts.

⊛ Rhus toxicodendron

- Indifference to family, but a dread of being alone.
- Cries while talking about the illness.
- Easily offended.
- Exhausted feelings, both physically and mentally.

⊛ Sepia

DOSAGE

USE THE 6C POTENCY. TAKE THREE TIMES A DAY, UNTIL AN IMPROVEMENT OCCURS. THEN CONSTANT REASSESSMENT IS NECESSARY AS RELAPSES ARE COMMON.

Fright

*F*right is the reaction to a sudden event that threatens you or someone close to you. If the feelings are sufficiently severe, it can be described as terror. You may be helped by choosing the medicine that best suits your symptoms.

SYMPTOMS / MEDICINE

- Marked palpitations.
- Fear that the cause of the fright was life threatening.

⊛ Aconitum napellus

- Anger after a fright.

⊛ Arnica montana

- Trembling and paralyzed feelings are experienced.
- An inability to face a challenge.

⊛ Gelsemium sempervirens

- A hysterical reaction to a fright is experienced.

⊛ Ignatia amara

- A tendency to collapse, is overwhelmed and apparently indifferent.
- Slow to answer.

⊛ Phosphoricum acidum

- Extremely sensitive and frightened by trifles.

⊛ Lycopodium clavatum

- Frightened by own imagination.
- Dizziness after a fright.

⊛ Opium *(prescription required in USA)*

- Oversensitive and easily startled.
- A great need for sympathy and company.

⊛ Phosphorus

- Anxious and sensitive to events.
- Feelings are made worse by consolation.

⊛ Silicea

DOSAGE

USE THE 30C POTENCY. TAKE A DOSE EVERY HALF HOUR FOR UP TO TEN DOSES.

Grief

Grief is the natural reaction to the loss of someone or something very important to you. The grieving process may take up to 18 months to complete, but if it lasts longer you may need professional help, including constitutional homeopathic treatment. If you find that your life is greatly disrupted by grief you should consider visiting a counselor to talk through what has happened because bottling it up can make it last longer.

SYMPTOMS/MEDICINE	
Early stages ❧ Shock because of sudden grief or loss. ❧ Mentally bruised by grief, a desire to be left alone.	⊛ Arnica montana
❧ Numb with grief. ❧ Fright because of the death of a loved one.	⊛ Opium *(prescription required in USA)*
Later stages ❧ Grief experienced by an idealistic person who is very sensitive. ❧ Alternating moods. ❧ Unable to come to terms with the loss.	⊛ Ignatia amara
❧ Nervous with fearful and insecure feelings. ❧ An aversion to being left on own. ❧ Wakes between 3 am and 5 am feeling anxious.	⊛ Kali carbonicum
❧ Weepy, depressed, and is averse to being comforted. ❧ Unresolved grief, or grief that was suppressed at the time of the loss.	⊛ Natrum muriaticum
❧ Profound nervous exhaustion and apathy. ❧ Unable to think or concentrate. ❧ Worse in the evening, and relief from fatigue is sought with sleep, but sleep is only fitful.	⊛ Phosphoricum acidum

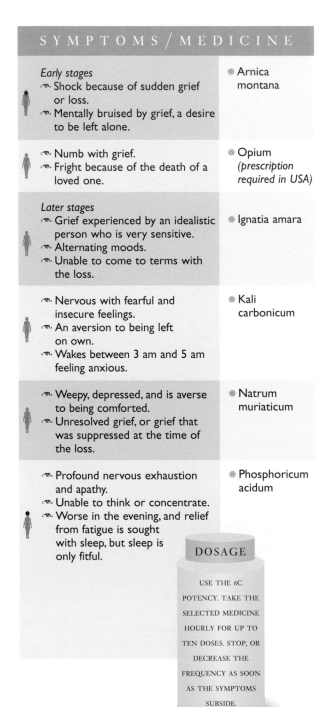

DOSAGE

USE THE 6C POTENCY. TAKE THE SELECTED MEDICINE HOURLY FOR UP TO TEN DOSES. STOP, OR DECREASE THE FREQUENCY AS SOON AS THE SYMPTOMS SUBSIDE.

Hypochondria

Hypochondria is the belief or fear that you have a serious illness, despite medical reassurance to the contrary. It can be a very disabling condition. Constitutional help from an experienced homeopath may be needed. See also Obsessions page 130.

Loneliness

Loneliness is the feeling of being isolated or abandoned. It is important to take steps to contact other people through social activities or voluntary work, but this is not easy because loneliness often leads to lack of confidence and depression (see page 125 and page 126).

Panic

Panic attacks are often irrational and unpredictable. It is a good idea to carry a homeopathic medicine that helps relieve the symptoms around with you so that you can take it as soon as you feel the symptoms coming on. (See also Fright and Phobias, page 127 and page 129).

DOSAGE

USE THE 30C POTENCY. TAKE EVERY HALF HOUR FOR UP TO TEN DOSES. STOP OR DECREASE THE FREQUENCY AS THE SYMPTOMS IMPROVE.

SYMPTOMS/MEDICINE	
❧ A fear of heights or of being in a crowded place. ❧ Great apprehension anticipating a stressful occasion, such as a driving test	⊛ Argentum nitricum
❧ Great anxiety and unease. ❧ Aversion to being left alone. ❧ Restlessness and inability to stay in one place.	⊛ Arsenicum album
❧ Trembling with anxiety, yet paralyzed. ❧ A desire to be held.	⊛ Gelsemium sempervirens

Mood swings

Changes of mood are normal and freely expressed by toddlers and adolescents but controlled by adults. More extreme mood changes are sometimes called mood swings. These tend to be a particular problem if you have a background of instability or unfairness in childhood, but some people seem to be prone to mood swings for genetic reasons. For women, of course, there is the added difficulty of hormonal changes (see Premenstrual syndrome, page 27). *If your mood changes are severe, you should consult your doctor.*

SYMPTOMS / MEDICINE

Symptoms	Medicine
Restless excitability, alternating with agitation and a conviction that death is imminent. Jealous feelings.	⊛ Apis mellifica
Time seems to pass too slowly, alternating with restless frustration.	⊛ Arsenicum album
Weakness and depression, alternating with restless impatience.	⊛ Calcarea carbonica
Periods of solitude and withdrawal alternating with spasms of excitement.	⊛ Nux vomica
Flashes of temper alternate with a desperate need for reassurance.	⊛ Phosphorus
Moods are constantly changing. A dependence on others alternating with anger and rage when criticized.	⊛ Pulsatilla

DOSAGE

USE THE 12C POTENCY. TAKE HOURLY FOR UP TO SIX DOSES.

HONEY BEE
(*APIS MELLIFICA*)

Phobias

Minor fears, which do not affect day-to-day living, are common and normal. They are dislikes rather than actual fears and can, if necessary, be overcome. Some people, however, have such a deep-seated fear, usually of a particular thing, that it disturbs their life and activities and can bring on actual physical symptoms. Listed below are some common medicines that can help reduce fear in general.

SYMPTOMS / MEDICINE

Symptoms	Medicine
Sudden panic. Great fear and anxiety. A fear of death but also fear of the future. Physical and mental restlessness is present.	⊛ Aconitum napellus
Apprehension before an event. Melancholia. A lack of self-confidence. Impulsive and wants to do things in a hurry. A desire for sweet things. Diarrhea comes on from fear.	⊛ Argentum nitricum
Fears loss of reason and misfortune. Apprehensive.	⊛ Calcarea carbonica
Emotional excitement and fear lead to bodily illness. Dull and listless. Stage fright and examination fears.	⊛ Gelsemium sempervirens
Fearful. Hates being left alone.	⊛ Kali carbonicum
Multiple phobias are experienced. Very sensitive.	⊛ Phosphorus
A fear of being alone and of the dark. Liking sympathy, may weep easily and be timid and irresolute.	⊛ Pulsatilla

DOSAGE

USE THE 30C POTENCY. TAKE EVERY 15 MINUTES UNTIL AN IMPROVEMENT IS MAINTAINED. IF TAKEN FOR A SPECIAL OCCASION, SUCH AS AN INTERVIEW, TAKE THREE DOSES ON THE DAY BEFORE, AND A FURTHER DOSE ON THE MORNING OF THE EVENT.

Obsessions

An obsession is a persistent and often irrational concern that may lead to normal actions, such as hand washing, being repeated so frequently as to be unreasonable. The following homeopathic medicines may help the condition but you may need a constitutional medicine to solve the problem.

If your symptoms are disrupting your life, consult your doctor, who may suggest behavioural therapy, which is often successful.

SYMPTOMS / MEDICINE

Symptoms	Medicine
☙ A preoccupation with death and dying. ☙ Feelings of utter worthlessness *(see your doctor urgently)*.	⊚ Aurum metallicum
☙ Recurrent fearful ideas about death or dying at a certain time. ☙ Irrational fears about the dark, shadows, crossing a road. ☙ Restlessness and agitation.	⊚ Aconitum napellus
☙ Feelings that the body and mind are separated, that the person is being controlled. ☙ Weak, exhausted and has poor memory and concentration.	⊚ Anacardium orientale
☙ Compulsive superstitious thinking. ☙ A fear of heart disease and cancer. ☙ Prone to sudden irrational impulses.	⊚ Argentum nitricum
☙ Violent, active and obsessional feelings. ☙ Fixed, rigid ideas and is angry and impatient. ☙ Face is often flushed and angry.	⊚ Belladonna
☙ Fear and anxiety, with a compulsion to do certain things. ☙ Unable to talk about emotions. ☙ Spasms and muscular cramps.	⊚ Cuprum metallicum
☙ Jealousy and suspicion, especially in sexual matters. ☙ Anger with self-doubt. ☙ A fear of heart disease or insanity.	⊚ Lachesis mutus
☙ A preoccupation with failure and an obsession with details. ☙ Feelings of futility and weakness. ☙ Oversensitive and chilly.	⊚ Silicea
☙ Mind is filled with all kinds of fears and speculation. ☙ A fear of disease, cancer, rejection and failure.	⊚ Sulphur
☙ Fixed fantastic ideas, such as feeling an animal in the abdomen or that the body is made of glass. ☙ Feels unattractive and worthless.	⊚ Thuja occidentalis

SULPHUR

DOSAGE

USE THE 30C POTENCY. TAKE EVERY TWO HOURS FOR UP TO SIX DOSES.

Shyness and timidity

*M*any people feel shy when meeting strangers, when initiating a conversation or simply when speaking in public. You may be prone to blushing and may even blush when you contemplate a situation that you will find embarrassing. In addition to trying some of the medicines described here you may find self-assertion classes helpful. Do not go out of your way to avoid situations that you think may embarrass you: the more you face up to the problem the easier it will be to overcome.

SYMPTOMS / MEDICINE

Symptoms	Medicine
➘ Intense shyness and prone to blush easily.	◉ Ambra grisea
➘ Sensitive and romantic. A useful remedy if fair haired.	◉ Cocculus indicus
➘ A dislike of company, but ill at ease alone and prone to depression.	◉ Conium maculatum
➘ Nervous, sensitive, flushes easily, even if anemic.	◉ Ferrum phosphoricum
➘ Apprehensive, despondent, indecisive and music leads to weeping. ➘ Feels the cold and may be prone to being overweight.	◉ Graphites
➘ Nervous, sensitive, with a tendency to overexcitement and weepiness, but efficient and learns quickly. ➘ Symptoms may change rapidly.	◉ Ignatia amara
➘ Slightest work seems impossible because of tiredness. ➘ Very nervous, easily startled and apt to lose control. ➘ Disinclined to talk, and irritable and tearful. ➘ Periods may be irregular, and may be pale.	◉ Kali phosphoricum
➘ Absent-minded, anxious, indolent and timid.	◉ Kali silicatum
➘ Melancholic feelings and a fear of being alone. ➘ Apprehensive and annoyed by trifles. ➘ Sensitive and may weep on being thanked. ➘ The worst time of day is 4–8 pm.	◉ Lycopodium clavatum
➘ Nervous, thin, irritable and very sensitive. ➘ Critical and easily offended.	◉ Nux vomica
➘ Oversensitive and very nervous. ➘ Restless, fidgety and cannot stand or sit still for long.	◉ Phosphorus
➘ Indecisive, rather laid back and gentle. ➘ Affectionate, mild and yielding. ➘ A tendency to weep easily.	◉ Pulsatilla
➘ Nervous, easily startled and is anxious about herself.	◉ Sabadilla
➘ Despondent, taciturn and ill humoured. ➘ Very sensitive and feels offended easily.	◉ Sarsaparilla
➘ Emotional sensitivity. ➘ Music causes weeping and trembling. ➘ Easily tired. ➘ May be prone to strange ideas such as being influenced by a superior power, or being pregnant when not.	◉ Thuja occidentalis

GRAPHITES

DOSAGE

USE THE 30C POTENCY. TAKE THREE TIMES A DAY FOR FOUR DAYS. REPEAT AT INTERVALS IF THE SYMPTOMS START TO RETURN.

Stress

DOSAGE

USE THE 12C POTENCY. TAKE THREE TIMES A DAY UNTIL THE SYMPTOMS ARE RELIEVED.

Stress results from a situation or event that disturbs your mental, emotional or physical health. In small amounts stress can be a stimulus, but if it is excessive or prolonged it can lead to a breakdown of health. Some suggestions to help you reduce the stress in your life are given on pages 118 and 119. Self-help homeopathic medicines will need to be chosen according to the symptoms that you are experiencing, such as depression, mood swings or temper (see pages 126, 129 and right).

To help you cope with stressful situations you may have come to rely on taking various substances, such as tea, coffee, alcohol, sugar and tobacco. The problem with relying on these substances too much is that you become accustomed to them, and tend to need greater amounts of them as time goes on.

SYMPTOMS / MEDICINE

Symptoms	Medicine
➤ A craving for tea. ➤ Withdrawal headaches and muscle pains.	◉ Thea
➤ A craving for coffee.	◉ Coffea cruda

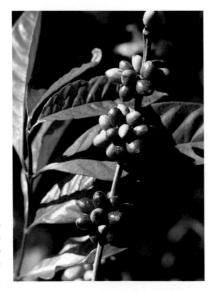

Coffea cruda, which is prepared from raw coffee berries, may help to relieve a craving for coffee.

Anger, temper, and irritability

Women vary in the way they react to annoying events or individuals. Indeed some are constantly angry due to real or imagined grievances. Others simply argue for the sake of arguing – it is part of their personality. However, irritability may be a feature of another illness – constant pain is one example. Worry can often show itself by outbursts of bad temper. Whatever the cause homeopathy will help.

SYMPTOMS / MEDICINE

Symptoms	Medicine
➤ Cannot bear to be touched or looked at. ➤ Anger occurs in many situations. ➤ Overexcitability.	◉ Antimonium crudum
➤ Anger follows a fright.	◉ Arnica montana
➤ Weakness and restlessness with exhaustion after the slightest exertion. ➤ Nightly aggravations. ➤ Anger, fear and worry.	◉ Arsenicum album
➤ Peevish at the least contradiction. ➤ Profound depression, perhaps with talk of suicide. ➤ Oversensitivity.	◉ Aurum metallicum
➤ Headache and dizziness from sitting up. ➤ Dry, parched mouth. ➤ Everything is irritating.	◉ Bryonia
➤ Absent-minded, and lacking in self-confidence.	◉ Calcarea silicata
➤ Anxiety and intolerance.	◉ Carboneum sulphuratum
➤ Wild anger, promiscuity and a tendency to swear.	◉ Cereus serpentinus
➤ Complains after a period of anger. ➤ Colic is often present. ➤ Anger causes perspiration.	◉ Chamomilla

- Nervous, with an aversion to being touched.
- Can get very angry, much worse at night.

⊛ Cina

- Abdominal pain after anger and with great indignation.

⊛ Colocynthis

- Laughs a lot.
- May be violent with anger and sorrow afterwards.

⊛ Crocus sativus

- Cannot bear the slightest contradiction.
- Feels much better if kept busy.

⊛ Helonias diocia

- Unreasonable anger.
- A headache follows the anger.
- Forever sighing and sobbing, with changeable moods.
- Melancholic and uncommunicative, symptoms may follow shocks, grief and disappointment.

⊛ Ignatia amara

- Very nervous and is easily startled.
- Pale, sensitive and weepy.

⊛ Kali phosphoricum

- Sudden anger with an impulse to do violence.

⊛ Mercurius solubilis

- Ill effects from anger with fear.

⊛ Natrum muriaticum

- Hateful, vindictive, headstrong but with hopeless despair.
- Sensitive to noise, pain and touch.

⊛ Nitricum acidum

- Violent temper and cannot bear contradiction.
- Generally irritable and angry.
- Anger from loud noises, which are painful.
- Anger may lead to indigestion.
- Irritable and cannot bear noise or smells.
- Sullen, fault-finding and with a fiery temperament.

⊛ Nux vomica

- A feeling that death is near.
- Irritable, easily offended and vexed at everything.

⊛ Petroleum

- Easily offended and indifferent to family.
- Very sad and weepy, with anxiety towards the evening.

⊛ Sepia

- Ill effects from anger and insults.
- Suppressed anger and indignation.

⊛ Staphysagria

- Feels depressed, weak, lazy and irritable.
- Selfish, with no regard for others.

⊛ Sulphur

- Sudden mood changes, and seems ungrateful and discontented.

⊛ Tarentula hispana

CUTTLEFISH
(*SEPIA*)

DOSAGE

USE THE 30C
POTENCY, TAKE
THREE TIMES A DAY
FOR FIVE DAYS

CHAPTER 10

EMERGENCIES

MEDICAL EMERGENCIES generally follow an accident or occur as a result of a sudden serious illness. Additionally, in family life, urgent relief is often needed for those illnesses that are not life-threatening but occur suddenly when immediate professional help is not available. Ideally, you should have a first-aid box at home that contains suitable homeopathic medicines for all these different types of emergency.

Immediately after accidents and the onset of sudden serious illnesses, your first priorities are to telephone for a doctor and/or an ambulance, and attend to the normal first-aid procedures. While you are waiting for professional help to arrive, however, there is much that you can do with a first-aid box that is stocked with well-chosen homeopathic medicines. This section of the book provides you with useful suggestions for a wide variety of emergencies. Both the victims and the onlookers may feel a sense of shock and one or more doses of Aconitum napellus in the highest potency you have available can be very helpful in combating their symptoms.

It is said that more people are converted to the use of homeopathy by Arnica montana than by any other homeopathic medicine. Arnica montana has an essential place in every first-aid box because of its effectiveness in treating both bruising and bleeding. Less well known, however, is its use during a suspected heart attack as it helps to allay anxiety, and to alleviate emotional or mental 'bruising' when you are left feeling very hurt or rejected after some disturbing conversation or event.

Less serious conditions, such as the sudden onset of diarrhea, vomiting, toothache or a sore throat usually respond well to starting the correct homeopathic medicine at the earliest opportunity. You will need to refer to the other sections contained in this book to choose the correct medicine.

ARNICA MONTANA

USING HOMEOPATHY IN AN EMERGENCY

❧ You can use any potency that you have available. The most easily available potencies, the 6c or the 30c, will provide quick relief, but using a higher potency is also safe. If you use the 6c potency you may find that you will have to repeat the dose more frequently and for longer.

❧ Homeopathic medicines can be used safely at the same time as conventional medicines and may even enhance their action.

❧ Once you have chosen the homeopathic medicine you should place it in the mouth of the patient as soon as possible.

❧ You can repeat the dose every five or ten minutes without risk, but once the condition of the patient is seen to be improving, you should not give a further dose until this effect appears to be wearing off.

❧ If there is no response after six doses you should consider changing the medicine.

YOUR FIRST-AID BOX

To start with, it is always a good idea to buy a few medicines specifically for emergencies and some suggestions for your basic first-aid box are given here. However, as you become more familiar with homeopathic medicines and begin to use them more for yourself and your family you will soon build up a store of homeopathic medicines, many of which can be useful to treat different ailments as they arise. Suggestions for the medicines that you are most likely to need for a more comprehensive first-aid box are given on the opposite page.

Homeopathic pills, granules and powders will keep indefinitely provided that they are stored in a cool dark place away from strong smells, including perfumes and mothballs. The tops of the bottles should be firmly tightened. Liquid potencies often have a short shelf life and the advice of your pharmacist should be sought.

AFTERCARE

Recovery time after an accident or serious injury can sometimes be shortened with homeopathic medicines, for example, Symphytum may aid the repair of a bone after a fracture. If you are using homeopathic medicines in this way you should tell your doctor.

Sometimes long-term symptoms seem to start at the time of an emergency, such as headaches after a head injury or panic attacks after a car accident. These can often be helped with homeopathic medicines but you may need to consult a homeopath for guidance to identify a remedy that will suit you.

FIRST AID

In addition to the normal contents of a first-aid box such as dressings, bandages and scissors you can keep a supply of homeopathic medicines for emergency use.

THE BASIC 15 REMEDIES

Shock, fright, angina, mastitis, sudden illness after being in a cold or draft.	*Aconitum napellus*
Insect stings, cystitis, rashes and swellings that are pink and shiny (like a bee sting).	*Apis mellifica*
Any injury where there is shock, bruising or angina.	*Arnica montana*
Diarrhea with vomiting, anxiety, colds and hay fever.	*Arsenicum album*
Sudden high fever, boils, heavy and painful periods.	*Belladonna*
Painful cough, influenza, mastitis, painful and swollen joints.	*Bryonia*
Frantic unbearable pain, for example earache or toothache.	*Chamomilla*
Low fevers accompanied by tiredness or hemorrhage.	*Ferrum phosphoricum*
Influenza that occurs with stage fright or before an ordeal such as an examination.	*Gelsemium sempervirens*
Nerve injuries, for example to the finger tips, toes, ears and base of the spine.	*Hypericum perforatum*
Grief, emotional shock, reactions to coffee or tobacco smoke.	*Ignatia amara*
Nausea, bronchitis and asthma.	*Ipecacuanha*
After too much food and/or alcohol, cystitis, hay fever, sudden colds or cramp.	*Nux vomica*
Nausea, vomiting, hormonal changes, period pains or styes.	*Pulsatilla*
Sprains and strains, chicken pox, shingles, cold sores or herpes.	*Rhus toxicodendron*

CREAMS

Cuts and sores	*Calendula/ Hypercal*
Bruises	*Arnica*
Sprains	*Ruta*
Burns	*Urtica urens* (cream or mother tincture)

A FURTHER 15 REMEDIES

Hay fever, colds tickling coughs.	*Allium cepa*
Fear anticipating such things as examinations or flying.	*Argentum nitricum*
Violent abdominal pains, for example periods or diarrhea, cramps.	*Colocynthis*
Sore eyes in colds and hay fever.	*Euphrasia officinalis*
Painful, festering boils and abscesses and puncture wounds.	*Hepar sulphuris calcareum*
Sinusitis.	*Kali bichromicum*
Puncture wounds, insect bites.	*Ledum palustre*
Anticipatory fears, digestive upsets or palpitations.	*Lycopodium clavatum*
Period pains, angina or colicky bowel pain.	*Magnesia phosphorica*
Sore throat or mouth ulcers.	*Mercurius solubilis*
Grief or rejection, premenstrual symptoms, colds and hay fever.	*Natrum muriaticum*
Digestive upsets, bronchitis, hemorrhage, sore throat or anxiety.	*Phosphorus*
Sprained ankles or wrists.	*Ruta graveolens*
Problems caused by changes in female hormone levels.	*Sepia*
Early morning diarrhea, anxiety, itchy skin conditions.	*Sulphur*

Bleeding

Hemorrhage

As well as homeopathic treatment, the necessary first-aid procedures should be carried out while waiting for medical assistance. *Always seek medical advice for unexplained, or severe, bleeding anywhere in the body.*

SYMPTOMS/MEDICINE

	Symptoms	Medicine
	❧ A sense of panic and great restlessness. ❧ A craving for ice-cold drinks.	◉ Aconitum napellus
	❧ For use after any form of injury, especially when there may be bruising.	◉ Arnica montana
	❧ Restlessness with anxiety and marked exhaustion.	◉ Arsenicum album
	❧ A loss of bright red blood occurs which clots easily. ❧ Head is hot; face is red.	◉ Belladonna
	❧ Patient shows signs of collapse with cold, clammy sweat. ❧ A steady seepage of dark-colored blood.	◉ Carbo vegetabilis
	❧ Faintness and weakness with ringing in the ears. ❧ The blood is dark, almost brown.	◉ Chinchona officinalis
	❧ The blood is profuse, bright red and clots easily. ❧ Especially useful for nosebleeds.	◉ Ferrum phosphoricum
	❧ A slow but steady flow of dark blood. ❧ Exhaustion, but no anxiety. ❧ Bleeding occurs from hemorrhoids.	◉ Hamamelis virginiana
	❧ The blood is bright red. ❧ Persistent bleeding, but in fits and starts. ❧ A feeling of emptiness in the stomach. ❧ A craving for ice-cold drinks.	◉ Phosphorus
	❧ A brisk flow of blood with dark clots and pelvic pain.	◉ Sabina

DOSAGE

USE THE 30C POTENCY. TAKE EVERY FIVE MINUTES UNTIL AN IMPROVEMENT IS MAINTAINED.

Cuts and lacerations

If the skin becomes damaged by being torn open, treatment to some extent depends upon the type of damage produced. When the cut is from a sharp blade, the result is known as an incised wound and it may bleed very freely because the damaged blood vessels cannot shut down easily. When the injury produces a wound with irregular edges, it is called a laceration. These tend to bleed less freely but are more likely to become infected. After cleaning with warm water, firm pressure or squeezing the edges of the wound together will usually stop the bleeding. A firm, clean dressing may then be put over the area.

SYMPTOMS/MEDICINE

	Symptoms	Medicine
	❧ For when there is immediate shock.	◉ Aconitum napellus
	❧ Good to use if there is a lot of bruising.	◉ Arnica montana
	❧ If there is much bleeding and infection is likely.	◉ Calendula officinalis
	❧ If the wound is deep and/or extensive, and if a lot of pain is being suffered.	◉ Hypericum perforatum

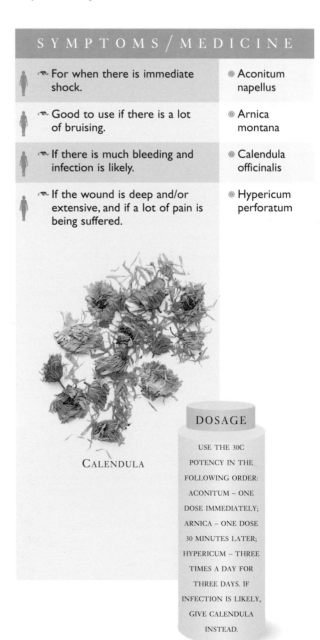

CALENDULA

DOSAGE

USE THE 30C POTENCY IN THE FOLLOWING ORDER: ACONITUM – ONE DOSE IMMEDIATELY; ARNICA – ONE DOSE 30 MINUTES LATER; HYPERICUM – THREE TIMES A DAY FOR THREE DAYS. IF INFECTION IS LIKELY, GIVE CALENDULA INSTEAD.

Insect bites and stings

*I*f the stinger is left in the skin, try to remove it carefully with tweezers, but do not squeeze it as the poison will be forced out into the skin. *If a sting occurs in the mouth or throat, or if there are multiple stings, go to a hospital at once.*

SYMPTOMS / MEDICINE

☜ For use as soon as possible after the sting occurs.	◉ Ledum palustre 30c – take one dose hourly for three doses.
☜ Where there is much burning, stinging and rapid swelling.	◉ Apis mellifica 30c – take one dose hourly for three doses.
☜ The area is red, hot and angry-looking.	◉ Cantharis 30c – take three times a day for four days.
☜ To treat a bee sting.	◉ Carbolicum acidum 30c – take one dose hourly for three doses.
☜ The area remains cold, numb and very sensitive, but is better after a cold dressing	◉ Ledum palustre 30c – take three times a day for four days.
☜ The area is hot and blue.	◉ Tarentula hispana 30c – take three times a day for three days.
☜ Where there is an itchy, blotchy, allergic type of skin reaction.	◉ Urtica urens 30c – take hourly until relief is obtained
☜ With a bee or wasp sting a few drops of the appropriate mother tincture dabbed on the area stung will help to soothe it.	◉ *Bee stings* – Urtica urens *Wasp stings* – Ledum palustre *Gnat bites* – Hypericum perforatum

Puncture wounds

*A*ny sharp object such as a nail, needle or garden fork can produce a puncture wound. If it is deep, there is considerable risk of infection having been introduced by the sharp object, and injury to deeper tissues may also have been caused. Puncture wounds require a tetanus injection.

SYMPTOMS / MEDICINE

☜ Use as soon as possible after the injury occurs.	◉ Ledum palustre 30c – take three times a day for two to three days.
☜ The wound still remains painful after treatment with Ledum palustre.	◉ Hypericum perforatum 6c – take three times a day for three to four days.
☜ The area remains cold and numb and is sensitive to touch, getting relief from cold applications.	◉ Ledum palustre 6c – take four times a day for four days.
☜ A splinter remains in the wound.	◉ Silicea 12c – take four times a days until it becomes removable.
☜ The area becomes infected, hot, red, swollen and painful.	◉ Hepar sulphuris calcarea 30c take three times a day for four days.

Burns, scalds and sunburn

*B*urns are injuries caused by heat, certain chemicals, electricity, extreme cold and radiation. When the heat is 'dry' the injury is called a burn; if the heat is 'moist', as in steam, the injury is known as a scald. The seriousness of the injury depends upon its size and also its depth.

A burn more than 2.5 cm/1 in square which goes deeper than the very surface of the skin needs medical attention. All but very small and minor burns and scalds require medical attention after immediate first-aid.

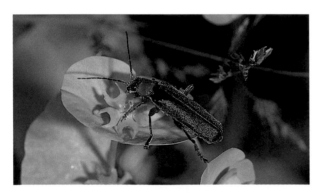

Cantharis, also known as the blister beetle, can ease the uncomfortable pain of blistered skin.

SYMPTOMS / MEDICINE

☞ There is always fright and shock.	◉ Aconitum napellus then Cantharis
☞ Where there is only minor redness of the skin.	◉ Urtica urens

DOSAGE

GIVE ACONITUM NAPELLUS, THE HIGHEST POTENCY, AVAILABLE AND THEN CANTHARIS 30C AT 15-MINUTE INTERVALS UNTIL THERE IS RELIEF.

DOSAGE

URTICA URENS 30C SHOULD BE GIVEN AT 30-MINUTE INTERVALS UNTIL RELIEF IS FELT. MOIST DRESSINGS OF URTICA URENS LOTION (15 DROPS OF MOTHER TINCTURE TO 250ML/9 FL OZ OF COLD, BOILED WATER) SHOULD BE PLACED ON THE AREA. THEN KEEP THE DRESSING MOIST AND LEFT UNDISTURBED.

Concussion and head injuries

*I*mmediate first-aid procedures should always be carried out. *All but minor bumps and bangs which may produce local tenderness and bruising require medical attention.* First give Arnica montana 30c and repeat at 15-minute intervals for three doses followed by Hypericum perforatum 30c every half-hour for four doses.

Fainting

*F*ainting is due to a temporary lack of oxygen to the brain. It can arise from being in a hot, stuffy atmosphere, or follow any sort of emotional upset or disturbance. *Frequent or repeated fainting attacks require medical investigation.*

SYMPTOMS / MEDICINE

☞ For after a fright or with severe pain.	◉ Aconitum napellus
☞ When anemia is present.	◉ Aceticum acidum
☞ If it occurs from overeating.	◉ Antimonium tartaricum
☞ If it comes about from fear, lack of breath and stomach ache.	◉ Arsenicum album
☞ If it happens on sitting up.	◉ Bryonia
☞ If it occurs because of stooping.	◉ Elaps corallinus
☞ If it happens after exertion.	◉ Glonoinum
☞ If it occurs from tight clothes.	◉ Lachesis mutus
☞ If it happens in a warm room.	◉ Lilium tigrinum
☞ If it occurs with hysteria and while eating.	◉ Moschus
☞ Fainting occurs from nasty smells.	◉ Nux vomica
☞ A tendency to faint.	◉ Sepia
☞ Occurs about 11 am.	◉ Sulphur
☞ Happens from the slightest exertion.	◉ Veratrum album

DOSAGE

USE THE 30C POTENCY. CRUSH A TABLET AND PLACE A FEW GRAINS ON THE TONGUE.

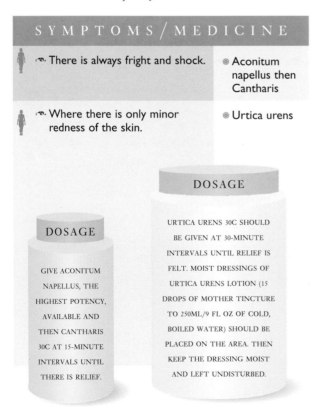

Heart attack

The symptoms of a heart attack are a sudden, agonizing, constricting chest pain, which may radiate to the neck, jaw or arms, mainly on the left side. The patient is usually in shock – cold and sweaty with a grey complexion and a shallow, rapid pulse. The pain does not pass with rest.

Sudden severe chest pain for which there is no apparent cause requires urgent diagnosis by a doctor as medical care is best started early. Homeopathic treatment and first-aid procedures should be applied while waiting for medical assistance.

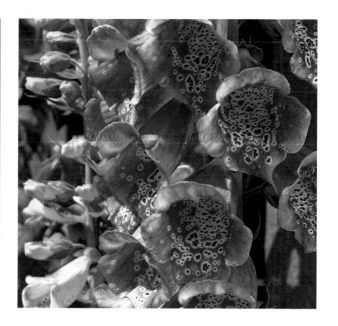

Digitalis, made from the foxglove, has been used to treat heart conditions for 2,000 years.

SYMPTOMS / MEDICINE

❧ Great anxiety with difficulty in breathing, plus numbness and tingling in the fingers. ❧ Feels better sitting up.	⊛ Aconitum napellus
❧ Chest pain after exertion or fatigue. ❧ Chest feels sore and bruised.	⊛ Arnica montana
❧ Heart feels as if grasped in a fist. ❧ Lower part of chest feels tied down and there are cries of pain.	⊛ Cactus grandiflorus
❧ Weakness and numbness in left arm. ❧ Skin has a blue tinge. ❧ Fears the heart will stop if move about.	⊛ Digitalis purpurea
❧ Wakes from sleep feeling smothered and unable to lie flat.	⊛ Lachesis mutus
❧ Violent pain in chest and left arm, pulse is very rapid and there is great difficulty in breathing.	⊛ Latrodectus mactans
❧ Woken by pain with heart feeling as if it is trapped in a vice. ❧ Need to bend double to try to ease the pain.	⊛ Lilium tigrinum
❧ Palpitations and irregular pulse, with paroxysms of suffocation and tightness across the upper chest.	⊛ Tabacum

DOSAGE

USE THE HIGHEST POTENCY YOU HAVE AND REPEAT AT FIVE-MINUTE INTERVALS UNTIL RELIEF IS OBTAINED.

Heatstroke

*E*xposure to high temperatures, particularly with high humidity, may lead to this condition. Early symptoms are headache, dizziness, nausea and lassitude. This may quickly lead on to muscle cramps, convulsions, collapse and coma. As well as using homeopathic treatment, first-aid procedures to cool the patient should be carried out. *Medical help is required.*

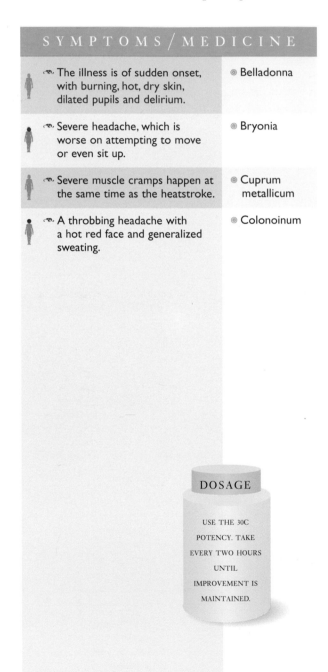

SYMPTOMS / MEDICINE	
↷ The illness is of sudden onset, with burning, hot, dry skin, dilated pupils and delirium.	⊛ Belladonna
↷ Severe headache, which is worse on attempting to move or even sit up.	⊛ Bryonia
↷ Severe muscle cramps happen at the same time as the heatstroke.	⊛ Cuprum metallicum
↷ A throbbing headache with a hot red face and generalized sweating.	⊛ Colonoinum

DOSAGE

USE THE 30C POTENCY. TAKE EVERY TWO HOURS UNTIL IMPROVEMENT IS MAINTAINED.

Stroke

*C*aused by a sudden cutting off of the blood supply to part of the brain, strokes vary according to the area involved and the amount of damage to the brain tissue. The symptoms can be anything from loss or diminution of muscle power in the affected part of the body to total coma and eventual death. *As well as using homeopathic treatment, first-aid procedures should be carried out while waiting for medical assistance.*

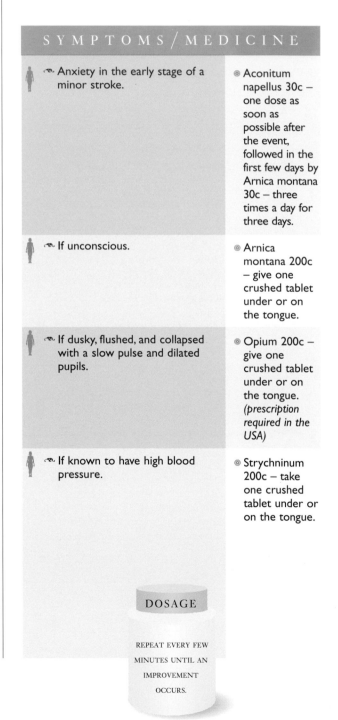

SYMPTOMS / MEDICINE	
↷ Anxiety in the early stage of a minor stroke.	⊛ Aconitum napellus 30c – one dose as soon as possible after the event, followed in the first few days by Arnica montana 30c – three times a day for three days.
↷ If unconscious.	⊛ Arnica montana 200c – give one crushed tablet under or on the tongue.
↷ If dusky, flushed, and collapsed with a slow pulse and dilated pupils.	⊛ Opium 200c – give one crushed tablet under or on the tongue. *(prescription required in the USA)*
↷ If known to have high blood pressure.	⊛ Strychninum 200c – take one crushed tablet under or on the tongue.

DOSAGE

REPEAT EVERY FEW MINUTES UNTIL AN IMPROVEMENT OCCURS.

Shock and collapse

Shock occurs after severe injuries, bleeding or burns and is due to the reduction in blood volume and blood pressure that these conditions produce. It may follow a nervous shock, such as a severe fright or the receipt of bad news. The symptoms occur because insufficient oxygen is carried to the nervous system and other tissues. The patient will have pale, cold, clammy, grey-colored skin, restlessness, shallow breathing and a weak pulse. In lesser shock the patient may just feel shaky for a few minutes or go into a faint.

As well as using homeopathic treatment, the necessary first-aid procedures should be carried out while waiting for medical assistance.

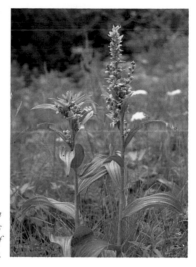

Veratum album, often used to treat shock, is prepared from the roots of the white false hellebore.

SYMPTOMS / MEDICINE

Symptoms	Medicine
❧ A sudden fright or shattering experience. ❧ Extreme terror, restlessness, rapid pulse and soaking sweat.	⊛ Aconitum napellus
❧ Trauma. ❧ Pale, panting and lacking a pulse. Either belittles the situation or feels that death is imminent.	⊛ Arnica montana
❧ Great restlessness and anxiety with a worried or even terrified expression. ❧ Pulse is weak or irregular. ❧ Lower eyelids appear to be puffy.	⊛ Arsenicum album
❧ Icy coldness with bluish, shrivelled-looking skin. ❧ Lips become drawn back, showing the teeth, and the voice is high-pitched or husky. ❧ Throws off the bedclothes. ❧ Eyes are upturned or closed.	⊛ Camphora
❧ Feels very cold, particularly about the knees.	⊛ Carbo vegetabilis
❧ Shock occurs after hemorrhage.	⊛ Chinchona officinalis
❧ Skin is cold and resembles marble. ❧ Beads of cold sweat appear on the forehead. ❧ Pale, drawn and sunken face. ❧ A feeble pulse. ❧ Watery saliva dribbles from mouth. ❧ Lips, hands and nails are blue.	⊛ Veratrum album

DOSAGE

REPEAT EVERY FEW MINUTES UNTIL IMPROVEMENT OCCURS.

Suffocation

*T*his condition occurs when the blood is unable to obtain sufficient oxygen due to some interference with respiration. The skin will have a purplish appearance and breathing may be irregular, eventually ceasing altogether. Possible causes include: obstruction of the air passages after choking or drowning; the tongue being swallowed while unconscious; the effects of drugs (including overdose) or electric shock; injuries to the chest wall; poisoning by carbon monoxide from car exhaust fumes if the victim is flushed.

First-aid procedures should be carried out while waiting for medical help. Once consciousness has been regained, homeopathic medicines may be administered.

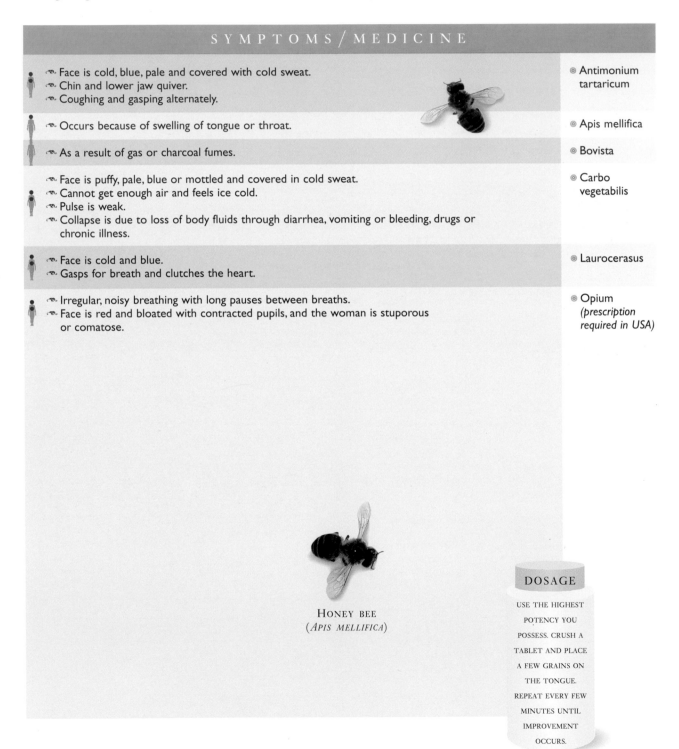

SYMPTOMS / MEDICINE

- ✒ Face is cold, blue, pale and covered with cold sweat.
- ✒ Chin and lower jaw quiver.
- ✒ Coughing and gasping alternately.

⊛ Antimonium tartaricum

- ✒ Occurs because of swelling of tongue or throat.

⊛ Apis mellifica

- ✒ As a result of gas or charcoal fumes.

⊛ Bovista

- ✒ Face is puffy, pale, blue or mottled and covered in cold sweat.
- ✒ Cannot get enough air and feels ice cold.
- ✒ Pulse is weak.
- ✒ Collapse is due to loss of body fluids through diarrhea, vomiting or bleeding, drugs or chronic illness.

⊛ Carbo vegetabilis

- ✒ Face is cold and blue.
- ✒ Gasps for breath and clutches the heart.

⊛ Laurocerasus

- ✒ Irregular, noisy breathing with long pauses between breaths.
- ✒ Face is red and bloated with contracted pupils, and the woman is stuporous or comatose.

⊛ Opium (prescription required in USA)

HONEY BEE
(*APIS MELLIFICA*)

DOSAGE

USE THE HIGHEST POTENCY YOU POSSESS. CRUSH A TABLET AND PLACE A FEW GRAINS ON THE TONGUE. REPEAT EVERY FEW MINUTES UNTIL IMPROVEMENT OCCURS.

Fractures

Broken bones

A fracture is a broken bone and the actual 'snap' of the bone may have been heard by the patient when it occurred. Depending on the site of the injury, there is usually pain which is increased by attempting to move the affected part. Swelling and tenderness develop, and in a bad fracture deformity of the affected part may be seen. First-aid treatment should be to prevent any movement of the fractured bone ends as this can lead to further damage and cause considerable pain and shock. *All fractures require hospital attention. Use first-aid procedures and homeopathic treatment as soon as possible after the injury is sustained.*

SYMPTOMS / MEDICINE

❧ Use as soon as possible for the pain and shock.	◉ Aconitum napellus 30c – one dose
❧ Suitable ten minutes after using Aconitum napellus, for bruising and soft tissue damage.	◉ Arnica montana 30c – four times a day for four days.
❧ Use after Arnica montana to aid bone union.	◉ Symphytum offincinale 12c – twice a day for two weeks.
❧ For use if healing and union are slow.	◉ Calcarea phosphorica 12c – twice a day for a further four to eight weeks.

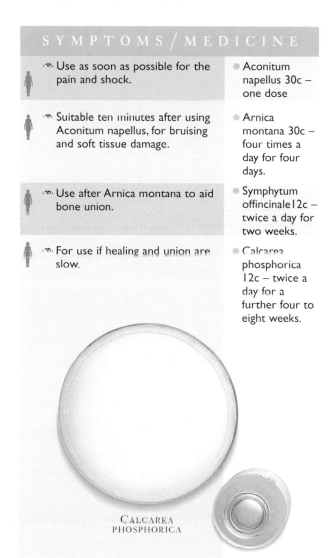

CALCAREA
PHOSPHORICA

Sprains and strains

A sprain occurs if the tissues around a joint are suddenly stretched or torn. There will be pain, tenderness and swelling, which are all increased by movement of the joint. A strain develops when a muscle is overstretched or torn by sudden violent movement and is diagnosed by the occurrence of a sudden sharp pain and swelling at the injury site. Both are sometimes difficult to distinguish from a fracture because of the large amount of damage caused. In these circumstances they should be treated as a fracture and the patient taken to a hospital. *All but minor sprains should have medical attention if they fail to improve after 24 hours or if the diagnosis is in doubt.*

SYMPTOMS / MEDICINE

❧ Initial bruising, swelling, pain and shock.	◉ Arnica montana 30c – take every hour for four doses, followed by Rhus toxicodendron 6c – four times a day until the symptoms are relieved.
❧ If the injury is close to a bony surface which is sore, use this medicine instead of Rhus tox.	◉ Ruta graveolens 6c – take four times a day until the symptoms are relieved.
❧ If the injury is close to a joint which has become swollen and painful on movement.	◉ Bryonia 30c – take three times a day for three days, followed by Rhus toxicodendron 6c – three times a day for three days.

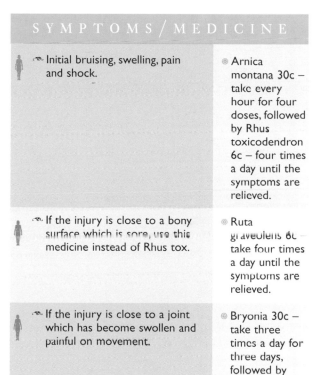

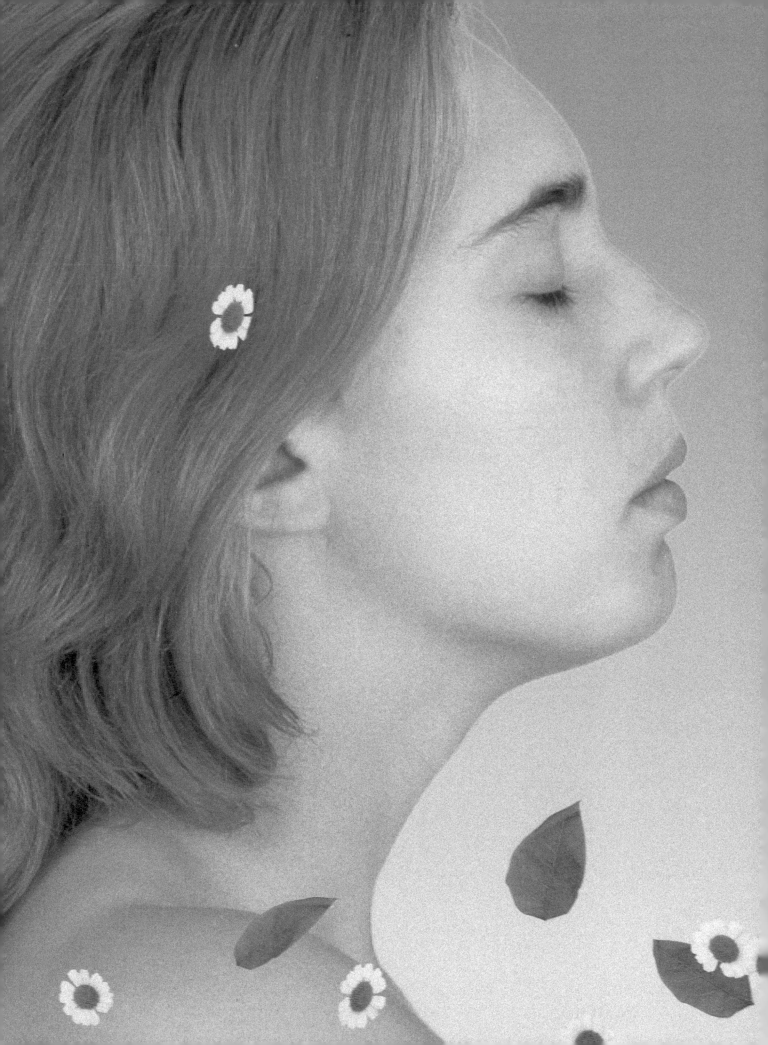

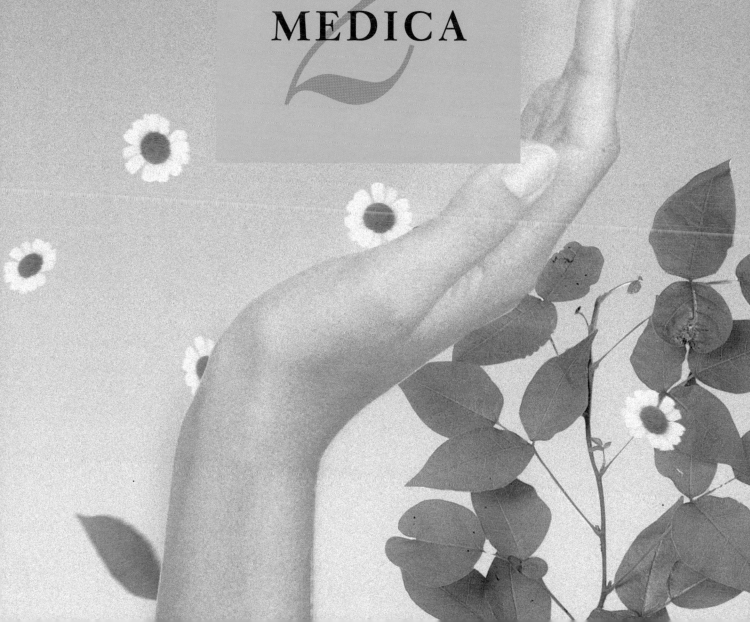

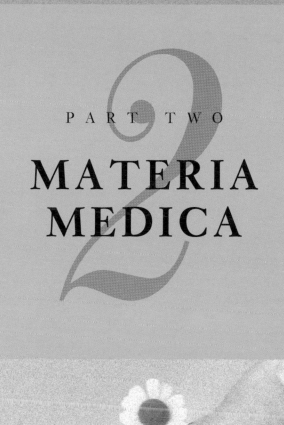

PART TWO

MATERIA
MEDICA

CHAPTER 11

COMMON HOMEOPATHIC MEDICINES

THE TERM *Materia Medica* is used by doctors to describe what is known about medicines and their uses. In homeopathy the term is used in a slightly different way to emphasize symptoms that are known to respond to the medicine being described, rather than the diagnosis. Different homeopathic medicines can be used to treat the same disease.

The *Materia Medica* section in this book provides more information about 50 of the medicines that are most frequently used in the homeopathic treatment of women. Use it to learn more about the medicine that you have selected after consulting Part 1 of the book.

For each medicine you will find a brief description of its source, together with further details as follows:

CONSTITUTIONAL AND PHYSICAL FEATURES

Some medicines seem to work best for people with particular physical features, or for ailments in a particular part of the body. Although these characteristics are briefly described in this section they do not have to be present for the medicine to work, particularly in acute illnesses. Conversely, if you find the constitutional and physical features describe you well, it may be that, for you, the medicine will help several ailments.

EMOTIONAL SYMPTOMS

Consider whether the characteristics described here fit you in general or in the way that you respond to your present symptoms or illness. In acute illnesses these symptoms are less important for your choice of medicine, but they can be helpful if you feel they describe your emotions.

PERSONAL CHARACTERISTICS

Homeopaths find these features helpful when they are deciding on a medicine. They may describe your present condition or reflect your usual likes and dislikes.

HOMEOPATHIC MEDICINES

- Homeopathic medicines usually come as pills or granules, which should be dissolved in the mouth, or as liquids which should be held in the mouth for a few minutes before being swallowed (see also page 11).
- The pills and granules are made of sugar, usually lactose (milk sugar), to which a medicinal solution has been added. If you are allergic to lactose or milk, a specialist homeopathic pharmacist may use another type of sugar, or suggest that you take a couple of drops of a solution containing the medicine.
- A few medicines are available as ointments or creams for application to the skin.
- Sometimes you will need a mother tincture so that you can dilute it yourself and use it for bathing the skin, gargling etc. Usually, you will need to add only about 10 drops to 250ml/½pt of water that has been boiled and cooled.
- If you only have pills available to give to a baby or unconscious person, crush one between two tablespoons and place in the mouth of your patient.

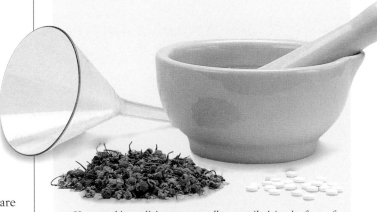

Homeopathic medicines are usually prescribed in the form of pills or granules made from sugar, which are medicated by adding a solution of the required medicine.

Aconitum napellus

*A*conitum napellus, *which is a very poisonous plant, is also known as monk's hood or wolf's bane. When you buy the homeopathic medicine derived from it you may find that it is simply known as Aconite.*

CONSTITUTIONAL AND PHYSICAL FEATURES *See pages 10–11*

Aconitum often suits women who are robust and lively when healthy, but who are unusually sensitive to pain. Women who develop a peculiar fear of death during pregnancy can also be helped by Aconitum.

> **MAIN USES**
> ❦ Conditions that occur suddenly, are often intense, and start after shock, or exposure to cold or wind.

EMOTIONAL SYMPTOMS

Most prominent reactions to any illness are acute anxiety and a mental and physical restlessness that make it impossible to keep still. There is a particular fear of death and maybe also a certainty of knowing exactly when you will die. Aconitum has a place in every homeopathic first-aid box; as a medicine for both the victim and the onlooker to ease anxiety after a shock, and to calm panic attacks.

PHYSICAL SYMPTOMS

Sensitive to pain, likely to cry out when in pain.

AILMENTS YOU CAN TREAT YOURSELF

In addition to those in chapters 1 to 10.

❦ **Conjunctivitis:** eyes and lids are red and feel hot; there are profuse tears and great intolerance of light.

❦ **Facial neuralgia:** usually left-sided, often with toothache and a hot, flushed face that becomes pale on sitting up.

PERSONAL CHARACTERISTICS

YOU FEEL WORSE:
❦ After exposure to wind, especially a cold, dry wind.
❦ In the evening.

YOU FEEL BETTER:
❦ For fresh air and resting.
❦ In the company of other people.

FOOD
❦ You have a great thirst especially for cold drinks.

FEARS
❦ You dislike being hemmed in, especially in a crowd.

Anacardium orientale

*T*he fruit from Semecarpus anacardium, *the marking nut tree, is the source of this medicine. It is made from the bitter juice contained in the pith that lies between the shell and the edible kernel.*

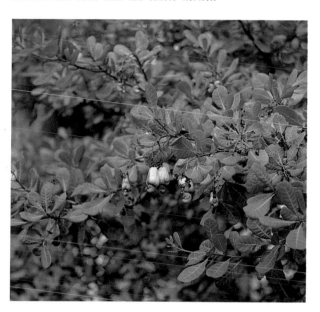

CONSTITUTIONAL AND PHYSICAL FEATURES *See pages 10–11*

People requiring Anacardium often have a deep-seated and intolerable mental conflict. As a result they feel inferior and will work hard to prove their worth, but they are sometimes callous or cruel. They tend to be overweight, as all their symptoms are improved by eating.

EMOTIONAL SYMPTOMS

Often lacking in self-confidence, and are unable to stop swearing, have a weak memory, and find making decisions difficult. Vivid nightmares may disturb sleep and leads to drowsiness during the day.

AILMENTS YOU CAN TREAT YOURSELF

See chapters 1 to 10.

> **MAIN USES**
> ❦ Digestive disorders.
> ❦ Skin conditions.
> ❦ Heart problems.

PERSONAL CHARACTERISTICS

YOU FEEL WORSE:
❦ In the cold.

YOU FEEL BETTER:
❦ After eating.

FEARS
❦ Of failure.
❦ That someone is behind you, or chasing you.

Apis mellifica

ften known as Apis, this medicine is prepared from the honey bee.

CONSTITUTIONAL AND PHYSICAL FEATURES *See pages 10–11*

Apis mellifica is indicated more frequently for women than men. The women most suited to it are busy, hard working and generally healthy, but they can be very irritable if crossed, and are protective of their families.

MAIN USES
🌾 Conditions affecting the skin, the mucous membranes (soft pink linings of the mouth, eyelids etc.) and the membranes that line the joints.

EMOTIONAL SYMPTOMS

May react to illness by becoming apathetic, weepy, hard to please, clumsy (may break things), and be drowsy or unable to concentrate at all.

AILMENTS YOU CAN TREAT YOURSELF
In addition to those in chapters 1 to 10.

🌾 **Headache:** a hot, heavy head with throbbing headache occurs that is relieved by pressure on the head.

🌾 **Cough:** a hoarse dry cough that is aggravated by lying down and after sleep, abdomen sore from coughing.

🌾 **Period problems:** periods late, irregular, accompanied by headaches.

🌾 **Rheumatism:** swollen, shiny, sensitive joints accompanied by stinging pains.

PERSONAL CHARACTERISTICS

YOU FEEL WORSE:
🌾 For heat, may faint entering a steam bath or sauna.
🌾 Around 3 pm.

YOU FEEL BETTER:
🌾 For exercise.
🌾 In the open air, after cool bathing.

FOOD
🌾 You are not thirsty, even with a high fever.

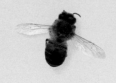

Argentum nitricum

he salt used to prepare this medicine is silver nitrate. It has been used in conventional medicine to remove unwanted skin lesions such as warts, as a dressing for infected skin wounds, such as burns, and also to prevent conjunctivitis in the newborn.

CONSTITUTIONAL AND PHYSICAL FEATURES *See pages 10–11*

Women who are likely to benefit from Argentum nitricum are outgoing and cheerful when well, but as they become less well they are prone to fears which they are unable to control. The anxiety can make them look older than their years. They have changeable emotions, and can be impetuous or suffer from impulsive thoughts or feelings that make them hurry, or want to do something silly, such as jumping from a high place. A feeling of physical weakness can be a recurrent problem, especially for women during the monthly period.

EMOTIONAL SYMPTOMS

Anxiety may already be present on waking and tend to cause tears and/or a fear of being left alone. In particular, there may be a worry about the seriousness of the illness, and a tendency to develop fixed ideas is difficult to get rid of, even though they seem silly.

AILMENTS YOU CAN TREAT YOURSELF
See chapters 1 to 10.

MAIN USES
🌾 Nervous disorders.
🌾 Digestive problems.

PERSONAL CHARACTERISTICS

YOU FEEL WORSE:
🌾 For the heat, but may be chilly if uncovered; need light covers.
🌾 After eating sweets, after anxiety or emotional events.
🌾 When anticipating a test, examination or interview.
🌾 For being alone.

YOU FEEL BETTER:
🌾 For being in cool air and for cold compresses.
🌾 In company.

FOOD
🌾 You have a craving for sweets, sugar and salt.

FEARS
🌾 Of being closed in.
🌾 Of high places.
🌾 Of diseases.
🌾 Of accidents.
🌾 Of being late.

Arnica montana

*A*rnica montana, *also known as leopard's bane or fall herb, grows at high altitudes and has long been used as a medicine by mountaineers after accidents.*

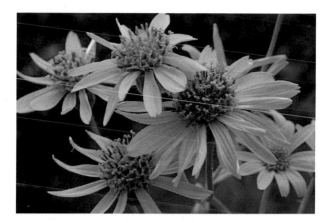

EMOTIONAL SYMPTOMS

Homeopaths recognize Arnica 'types' as women who deny that anything is wrong with them when they are ill, and want to be left alone. They tend to be nervous, despondent, morose and oversensitive, often complaining that the bed and pillow are too hard. However, you do not have to have these symptoms to benefit from Arnica.

> **MAIN USES**
> ⚘ Providing relief for physical injury, and soothing mental 'bruising'.

AILMENTS YOU CAN TREAT YOURSELF

In addition to those in chapters 1 to 10.

⚘ **Fatigue:** travel fatigue, jet lag, an emotional reaction after having had an accident.

⚘ **Muscular pains:** after exertion, such as gardening or childbirth; can be avoided by taking a dose beforehand, and repeating it when needed.

PERSONAL CHARACTERISTICS

YOU FEEL WORSE:
⚘ From touch or movement.
⚘ In the evening and night.

YOU FEEL BETTER:
⚘ For clear, cold stimulating weather.
⚘ Lying down with your head low.

Arsenicum album

*C*ommonly known as white arsenic, arsenic trioxide is the source of this medicine. Other arsenic salts are used in homeopathy but this is the most important and may simply be called 'Arsenicum'.

CONSTITUTIONAL AND PHYSICAL FEATURES

See pages 10–11

Arsenicum album best suits anxious, restless women with a great desire for order: they are extremely tidy and clean, conservative in their outlook, plan all enterprises carefully, and are careful about money, even to the point of stinginess. They are prone to fears, particularly about their health, and need much support from family and friends. Any pain is usually described as 'burning' but can be helped by warmth.

> **MAIN USES**
> ⚘ As a constitutional medicine, but particularly for problems affecting the digestive system and the skin.

EMOTIONAL SYMPTOMS

Being ill can be a source of anxiety in itself and any tendency to be anxious is more difficult to control than usual. May believe that the illness is serious, even though the doctor is reassuring, and may even despair of recovery. These worries sometimes extend to family and friends and there is a tendency to fear for their safety and well-being. These symptoms are more severe for Arsenicum 'types'.

PHYSICAL SYMPTOMS

Discharges (from ears, eyes, nose, vagina, anus) occur that have a burning feeling on the skin.

AILMENTS YOU CAN TREAT YOURSELF

In addition to those in chapters 1 to 10.

⚘ **Conjunctivitis:** inflamed eyes, sensitive to light, and swollen lids that can become red and scaly.

⚘ **Dandruff and scalp irritation:** severe irritation with hair loss in circular patches.

⚘ **Sore throat:** burning pain sometimes relieved by warm drinks; a feeling of constriction making swallowing difficult; sometimes burning painful ulcers.

PERSONAL CHARACTERISTICS

YOU FEEL WORSE:
⚘ In cold weather.
⚘ Between midnight and 2 am.
⚘ For being alone.
⚘ At sea.

YOU FEEL BETTER:
⚘ For being warm (but like head in fresh air during illness).
⚘ For moving about.

FOOD
⚘ A thirst for frequent small drinks.
⚘ Fat, sour food and alcohol is desired.
⚘ An aversion to grains, peas and beans.

FEARS
⚘ Of death.
⚘ Of cancer.

Aurum metallicum

This medicine is made from metallic gold and is often known simply as Aurum even though other gold salts are occasionally used in homeopathy.

CONSTITUTIONAL AND PHYSICAL FEATURES *See pages 10–11*

Aurum metallicum is best suited to women who are very idealistic and set themselves very high standards: they often hold strong religious beliefs. When they fail to achieve their goals, for whatever reason, or suffer bereavement or disappointment in affairs of the heart, they may react first with anger but are then often plunged into deep depression. They are also prone to addictive behaviour such as alcoholism or drug abuse, and hate to be contradicted.

EMOTIONAL SYMPTOMS

The most frequent reaction to adverse circumstances is deep depression for which medical advice should certainly be sought and Aurum metallicum should only be taken with the doctor's agreement. However, less severe depression, especially when anger is felt, or in winter, will often be eased by Aurum metallicum.

AILMENTS YOU CAN TREAT YOURSELF

In addition to those in chapters 1 to 10.

❧ **Arthritis:** rheumatic pains that wander from joint to joint and which are worse at night.

❧ **Headaches:** violent pain, causing a feeling of confusion. They are worse at night.

❧ **Heart symptoms:** palpitations especially after exertion or emotional events. Feeling as if heart has stopped, followed by thumping sensation.

❧ **Sinusitis:** with a blocked up nose, sometimes with small ulcers inside. Pain around the root of the nose especially on the right side.

PERSONAL CHARACTERISTICS

YOU FEEL WORSE:
❧ For emotional disturbance and mental exertion.
❧ For cold weather, cloudy weather, winter.
❧ During the night.

YOU FEEL BETTER:
❧ For music.
❧ In the open air.

FOOD
❧ A desire for milk coffee, alcohol, sweets.
❧ A strong aversion to meat.

FEARS
❧ Of failure.
❧ Of high places.
❧ Of heart disease.

SLEEP
❧ May wake after three to four hours of sleep moaning or crying out.

MAIN USES
❧ Depression, headaches, sinusitis, and heart disease.

Belladonna

Atropa belladonna is commonly known as deadly nightshade. It is the source of several medicines used in conventional medicine. Homeopathic Belladonna is prepared from the whole plant, which is harvested as it starts to flower.

CONSTITUTIONAL AND PHYSICAL FEATURES *See pages 10–11*

In health, those best suited to Belladonna are lively, sensitive, pleasant women, but they are prone to illnesses with sudden onset, often after suffering a change in temperature, such as being chilled or overheated. More chronic conditions have a slower onset. Belladonna can also help anyone who has a sudden feverish illness or area of inflammation, such as a boil, tonsillitis or ear infection. Typically, the patient is flushed, with widely dilated pupils and pain that throbs with every heartbeat, but the hands and feet may be cold.

MAIN USES
❧ In the very early stages of an acute feverish illness, but also has wider constitutional use.

EMOTIONAL SYMPTOMS

Likely to respond to any kind of disturbance with anger and may even become violent. When there is a fever, there may also be delirium, possibly with hallucinations.

AILMENTS YOU CAN TREAT YOURSELF *In addition to those in chapters 1 to 10.*

❧ **Arthritis:** hot swollen joints. Pain is worse for being jarred or touched.

❧ **Abdominal pain:** with distension, worse for touch, even the weight of the bedclothes irritates, and nausea or vomiting.

❧ **Facial neuralgia:** burning pain in the face, which is flushed with twitching muscles.

❧ **Headaches:** severe, congestive, throbbing pain in the front of head, made worse by lying down with head low, from light, noise, or being jarred. Pain is often relieved by firm pressure and applying cold applications.

PERSONAL CHARACTERISTICS

YOU FEEL WORSE:
❧ For being touched.
❧ For noise.
❧ In the afternoon.
❧ For any change in temperature.

YOU FEEL BETTER:
❧ When lying down with the head raised.

FOOD
❧ Either not thirsty or dread a drink.
❧ A craving for lemony foods.

SLEEP
❧ Lying on abdomen.
❧ May be disturbed.
❧ May dream of falling.

Berberis vulgaris

This medicine is prepared from the roots of Berberis vulgaris, *which is also known as common barberry, or pipperidge bush.*

CONSTITUTIONAL AND PHYSICAL FEATURES *See pages 10–11*

Berberis is not used very frequently, but those who need it often feel tired out and apathetic, with little stamina. Any pains tend to move around the body and often radiate from one point.

AILMENTS YOU CAN TREAT YOURSELF

In addition to those in chapters 1 to 10.

- **Arthritis:** pains that radiate from the affected joint and/or move from joint to joint.
- **Gallstone colic:** (in addition to conventional treatment) pain aggravated by pressure.

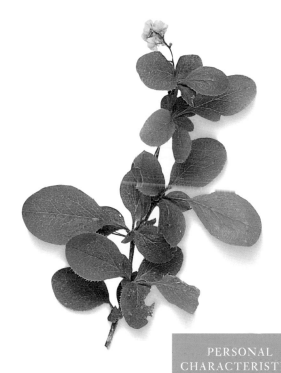

PERSONAL CHARACTERISTICS

YOU FEEL WORSE:
- From movement, stepping hard or jarring.

YOU FEEL BETTER:
- From being in the open air.
- After urination.

MAIN USES
- Infections in the urinary system, skin and joint conditions.

Bryonia

Bryonia alba, or white bryony, is a climbing plant that grows in hedgerows and sometimes develops a huge root weighing several pounds. The homeopathic medicine is made from the root that is harvested just before the plant flowers.

CONSTITUTIONAL AND PHYSICAL FEATURES
See pages 10–11

People needing Bryonia as a constitutional medicine are often in business and work hard to avoid financial problems and poverty. They tend to be rather irritable and fall ill after anger or disappointment. However, many people who are not at all like this also benefit from Bryonia, particularly for acute illnesses, and it is important to consider the likes and dislikes. A leading indication is pain that is made worse by any movement but is usually relieved by pressure. As a result, the patient wants to keep still, may lie on the painful side and prefers not to be disturbed. A dry mouth and thirst are also common symptoms.

MAIN USES
- Acute illnesses and rheumatism, but also has wider constitutional use.

EMOTIONAL SYMPTOMS:

Bad tempered, irritable and, most of all, want to be left alone. Prefer not to talk and find enquiries about what is wrong, even from the doctor, very annoying. If running a high fever, may feel confused and believe that are away from home, which is where you want to be.

AILMENTS YOU CAN TREAT YOURSELF

In addition to those in chapters 1 to 10.

- **Arthritis and backache:** red, swollen hot joints with stitching pain that is made worse by movement.
- **Diarrhea:** in hot weather, after cold drinks when overheated, worst in the morning, after getting up or moving about.
- **Headaches:** a bursting pain, usually on one side, starts in the front and extends to base of skull, worse for any movement including just moving the eyes.

PERSONAL CHARACTERISTICS

YOU FEEL WORSE:
- When cold, in cold weather or cold wind, or from getting hot.
- At around 9 pm.
- On waking.

YOU FEEL BETTER:
- For lying on the painful side and from pressure.
- After perspiring.

FOOD
- A desire for infrequent cold drinks.

SLEEP
- Usually on left side.

Calcarea carbonica

This medicine was first prepared by Hahnemann himself using the middle layer of an oyster shell. The same source of calcium carbonate is used today.

CONSTITUTIONAL AND PHYSICAL FEATURES *See pages 10–11*

Typical Calcarea carbonica women are very hard working, responsible and conscientious, but they are apt to take on too much and become overwhelmed.

A lack of stamina means they are more likely to be methodical plodders rather than brilliant achievers, and their timidity usually means they dislike being in the limelight. They tend to be obstinate, rather pessimistic and fear serious illness, and can be forgetful and confused. Nightmares or night terrors can be a problem. Calcarea carbonica 'types' are often fair-skinned, blue eyed and tend towards obesity, even on a low-calorie diet. However, many other people benefit from this medicine.

EMOTIONAL SYMPTOMS

Mental (and physical) exhaustion often cause health to break down leading to loss of interest in everything and become depressed, and even despair of recovery. Also likely to be troubled by the loss of security that can come with illness and also dislike hearing bad news.

AILMENTS YOU CAN TREAT YOURSELF

In addition to those in chapters 1 to 10.

❧ **Colds:** frequent, may have ongoing catarrh and nasal obstruction, and recurring enlarged neck glands.

❧ **Cough:** tickly, worse at night or after eating.

❧ **Headaches:** after exertion, during the menstrual period. They may be accompanied by nausea and an intolerance to light.

> MAIN USES
> ❧ As a constitutional medicine.

PERSONAL CHARACTERISTICS

YOU FEEL WORSE:
❧ In cold wet weather.
❧ For overexertion, especially walking uphill or climbing stairs.
❧ From getting wet.

YOU FEEL BETTER:
❧ In a dry climate.
❧ When constipated.

FOOD
❧ You have a craving for eggs; sweets; salt and indigestible items such as chalk and dirt.
❧ An aversion to fat, meat and coffee.

FEARS
❧ Of high places (even for someone else).
❧ Of mice and rats.
❧ Of going mad.
❧ Of poverty.
❧ Of serious illness.
❧ Of storms.

PERSPIRATION
❧ Cold, damp hands and feet; feet become hot and sweaty in bedsocks; also a perspiring head, especially at night.

Calcarea phosphorica

Dilute phosphoric acid is added to lime water to make the calcium phosphate used for this medicine.

CONSTITUTIONAL AND PHYSICAL FEATURES
See pages 10–11

Deep-seated discontentment marks the personality of the Calcarea phosphorica type, yet they can be open, friendly and sensitive when well. They are easily bored and have a strong desire to travel.

EMOTIONAL SYMPTOMS

An inability to describe the complaint exactly but feel dissatisfied and discontented. Symptoms feel much worse when thought about.

AILMENTS YOU CAN TREAT YOURSELF

In addition to those in chapter 1 to 10.

❧ **Digestive system:** colicky pain when eating, sometimes with diarrhea. Abdominal distension relieved by belching.

❧ **Arthritic pains:** in neck and joints, made worse by cold and drafts.

> MAIN USES
> ❧ As a constitutional medicine.

PERSONAL CHARACTERISTICS

YOU FEEL WORSE:
❧ In damp conditions, especially when the snow is melting.
❧ In drafts.

YOU FEEL BETTER:
❧ In warm dry weather.

FOOD
❧ Great hunger and thirst.
❧ There is a craving for bacon, ham, salt or smoked meats.

FEARS
❧ Of thunderstorms.
❧ Of the dark.

Cantharis

This medicine is pre-pared from an insect known as the Spanish fly or blister beetle. It contains an irritant chemical that can blister the skin.

> ### MAIN USES
> ❧ Conditions affecting the urinary system and the skin.

EMOTIONAL SYMPTOMS

There is a tendency to react to pains, which often start suddenly and are burning and severe, with frantic anger.

AILMENTS YOU CAN TREAT YOURSELF

In addition to those in chapters 1 to 10.

❧ **Diarrhea:** with burning stools that are very painful to pass and may contain blood.

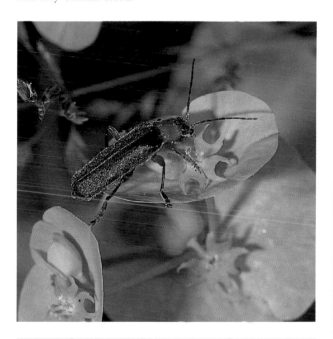

PERSONAL CHARACTERISTICS

YOU FEEL WORSE:
❧ Before urinating.
❧ At the sight or sound of water.
❧ For being touched.

YOU FEEL BETTER:
❧ When warm.
❧ For resting quietly in the dark.

FOOD
❧ A burning thirst, but an aversion to drinking.

FEAR
❧ Of mirrors.

Carbo vegetabilis

This medicine is prepared from vegetable charcoal. In conventional medicine charcoal is taken internally to absorb intestinal gas. It is also used externally as a deodorant for offensive wounds.

CONSTITUTIONAL AND PHYSICAL FEATURES

See pages 10–11

The typical Carbo vegetabilis 'type' is sluggish, obese, lazy and feels chilly, but the medicine is probably more often used for conditions in which the body is weak from debilitating illnesses, such as prolonged diarrhea or after taking drugs, and/or when the digestive system is weak. A collapsed state can sometimes develop when the patient, whose skin is cold, sweaty and may have a mottled appearance, demands an open window or a fan. Homeopaths sometimes call Carbo vegetabilis the 'corpse reviver' as it has a well-known ability to revive collapsed, unconscious people, especially the elderly.

> ### MAIN USES
> ❧ For digestive disorders, collapsed and weak states.

PERSONAL CHARACTERISTICS

YOU FEEL WORSE:
❧ When covered up, despite being cold.
❧ After rich food.

YOU FEEL BETTER:
❧ For moving fresh air, even when you are cold.
❧ After belching.

FOOD
❧ A craving for sweets and salt.
❧ An aversion to rich fatty food and meat.

FEARS
❧ Of ghosts; the dark.

EMOTIONAL SYMPTOMS

Although there may be a feeling of weakness and aversion to mental effort, there may also be feelings of hurt and irritation if the condition is not fully appreciated by those looking after you. May long for some excitement, believing that it will help to overcome the illness, but as the illness progresses, may still be overcome by physical weakness.

AILMENTS YOU CAN TREAT YOURSELF

In addition to those in chapters 1 to 10.

❧ **Chest symptoms:** shortage of breath with rattling mucus, a feeling of suffocation and anxiety; symptoms are sometimes caused by overeating or accompanied by abdominal distension and wind; may need to sit up in bed and want moving air from a window or a fan.

❧ **Chilblains:** on the toes, which become red and swollen.

❧ **Cramp:** especially on the soles of feet; legs feel heavy and numb; coldness from the knees down.

Caulophyllum thalictroides

This medicine is made from Caulophyllum thalictroides, *known as blue cohosh.*

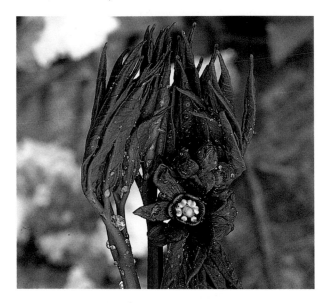

PHYSICAL FEATURES

Caulophyllum restores or enhances muscle tone in the walls of the uterus (womb). It is also useful for arthritis that is confined to the small joints, especially those of the hands.

EMOTIONAL SYMPTOMS

May feel exhausted and/or experience an inner trembling and anxiety.

AILMENTS YOU CAN TREAT YOURSELF

In addition to those in chapters 1 to 10.

❧ **Arthritis:** joint pains in the hands and toes that come and go every few minutes; stiffness of affected joints.

PERSONAL CHARACTERISTICS

YOU FEEL WORSE:
❧ During pregnancy.
❧ When period is delayed.
❧ After coffee.

YOU FEEL BETTER:
❧ When warmly dressed.

MAIN USES
❧ For conditions affecting the uterus (womb), arthritis of the small joints.

Causticum

Hahnemann himself devised the preparation of this medicine, which is unique to homeopathy, from equal parts of slaked lime (calcium hydroxide) and potassium bisulphate.

CONSTITUTIONAL AND PHYSICAL FEATURES

See pages 10–11

Women who need Causticum have repeatedly suffered grief and, sometimes as a result, developed a strong personality. Not only do they want to be in charge of their own lives but they also have a well developed sense of justice, may be politically active and display a tendency to exaggerate. At the same time they can be exceedingly sensitive and sympathetic to the suffering of others. Physically they are often lean, may have dark hair and eyes and a sallow skin.

EMOTIONAL SYMPTOMS

May feel mentally dull and fatigued or forgetful, and needing to check and double-check that have done things, for example, lock the door. Feel deeply for other people and may avoid listening to the news when it portrays any kind of suffering. Can be prone to feeling hurried.

AILMENTS YOU CAN TREAT YOURSELF

In addition to those in chapters 1 to 10.

❧ **Eye conditions:** when you have a cold, upper lids may feel heavy, or weak and paralyzed, and may close them involuntarily; may produce stinging tears.

❧ **Facial neuralgia** or paralysis (Bell's palsy): usually on the right after exposure to cold wind.

❧ **Rheumatic conditions:** pains may feel tearing and can be made worse by cold, overuse or dry weather; restless legs that occur at night; tendons may seem contracted.

❧ **Throat** desire to clear throat, cough to clear mucus.

MAIN USES
❧ As a constitutional medicine, and for conditions affecting the nervous system, joints and muscles.

PERSONAL CHARACTERISTICS

YOU FEEL WORSE:
❧ When cold or exposed to drafts.
❧ Around 4 pm or dusk.
❧ For the motion of travelling.

YOU FEEL BETTER:
❧ In cloudy or wet weather.
❧ After a cold drink.

FOOD
❧ A desire for salt, bacon, smoked meat, cheese and eggs.
❧ Either a desire for or aversion to sweets or fish.

FEARS
❧ Of the dark.
❧ Of animals, especially dogs.
❧ 'That something bad will happen'.

Chamomilla

German or wild chamomile is the plant that is used to prepare this medicine.

AILMENTS YOU CAN TREAT YOURSELF

In addition to chapters 1 to 10.

❧ **Toothache and earache:** especially if one cheek is flushed and the other one is pale.

❧ **Arthritic pains:** worse at night in a warm bed, but are relieved by walking about.

❧ **Withdrawal symptoms:** following abuse of coffee or of drugs.

PERSONAL CHARACTERISTICS

FEEL WORSE:
❧ For being touched.
❧ Around 9 pm.
❧ Going out in the wind.

FEEL BETTER:
❧ For putting feet out of bed at night.

FOOD:
❧ You have a thirst for cold drinks.

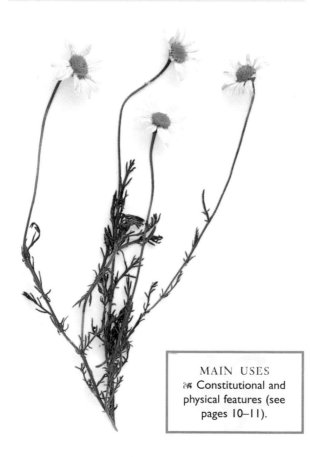

MAIN USES
❧ Constitutional and physical features (see pages 10–11).

Chinchona officinalis

You may find this medicine is sold as Cinchona. It is prepared from the bark of the quinquina tree, which is native to the eastern slopes of the Andes. It was introduced into Europe as a fever medicine by the Jesuits, and has also been known as Jesuit powder or Peruvian bark.

MAIN USES
❧ Digestive problems.
❧ Migraines.

CONSTITUTIONAL AND PHYSICAL FEATURES
See pages 10–11

Chinchona officinalis has long been used for recurrent fevers or when health has been slow to return following the loss of a body fluid through as diarrhea or hemorrhage. With modern medical care these situations are less common, but Chinchona officinalis is still useful for delayed convalescence. The type of woman most likely to respond to it is idealistic and sensitive to criticism.

EMOTIONAL SYMPTOMS

May feel irritable, suffer unpredictable moods and dislike any noise.

AILMENTS YOU CAN TREAT YOURSELF

In addition to those in chapters 1 to 10.

❧ **Digestive disorders:** abdominal distension and bloating; gallbladder colic (in addition to conventional treatment); painless diarrhea, which may follow after eating fish, fruit or drinking milk.

❧ **Fever:** that recurs, especially if there is a history of malaria.

❧ **Headache:** neuralgic pain relieved by firm pressure, may recur alternate days or every seventh day: sometimes associated with gallbladder or liver disorders, and/or with a bitter taste in the mouth.

❧ **Skin:** may be sensitive or painful during a fever; scalp may be sensitive to being brushed.

PERSONAL CHARACTERISTICS

YOU FEEL WORSE:
❧ For being touched.
❧ In foggy or cold damp weather.
❧ In the autumn.
❧ After any discharge, such as diarrhea or pus.

YOU FEEL BETTER:
❧ When any painful areas are pressed hard or firmly held.

FOOD
❧ A desire for sweets and salt.
❧ An aversion to hot food, fruit and fat.

FEARS
❧ Of night time.
❧ Of animals and dogs.

FEARS
❧ Of suffering night sweats.

Cimicifuga racemosa

This plant is found in North America where it is commonly known as black cohosh, bugbane or black snake root. It was originally used in a medicinal way by the Indian tribes.

CONSTITUTIONAL AND PHYSICAL FEATURES *See pages 10–11*

Women needing Cimicifuga racemosa are often extroverted, excitable and talkative, possess a vivid imagination and are also prone to phobias.

EMOTIONAL SYMPTOMS

You become depressed very easily when you are ill or when things go wrong.

AILMENTS YOU CAN TREAT YOURSELF

In addition to those in chapters 1 to 10.

❧ **Neck and back:** muscular neuralgic pain occurs affecting the neck and/or some small spinal muscles causing stiffness.

❧ **Extremities:** rheumatic pains are felt in muscles; pains occur that move, and are made worse by cold damp weather.

❧ **Headaches:** either at the back of head or coming from neck and shoulders; can be severe and may also have a stiff neck; may feel the top of the head might fly off.

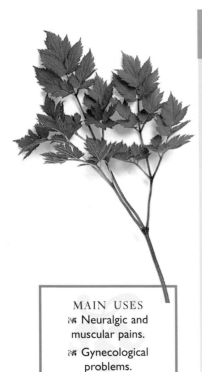

PERSONAL CHARACTERISTICS

YOU FEEL WORSE:
❧ During a period, the heavier it is the worse you feel.
❧ In damp cold air.
❧ After a change in the weather.

YOU FEEL BETTER:
❧ When warmly wrapped up.
❧ For moving about.
❧ After eating.

FEARS
❧ Of insanity.
❧ Of death or being murdered.

MAIN USES
❧ Neuralgic and muscular pains.
❧ Gynecological problems.

Colocynthis

This medicine is often called Colocynth and it is prepared from Citrullus colocynthis, *commonly known as bitter cucumber or bitter apple.*

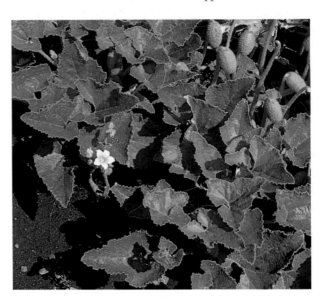

CONSTITUTIONAL AND PHYSICAL FEATURES *See pages 10–11*

Colocynth is best suited to rather reserved, conservative people with strong views on what is correct. They are easily angered or made indignant by contradiction, especially if they feel put down, and tend to develop various neuralgias and colicky pains as a result.

EMOTIONAL SYMPTOMS

Anger and indignation.

AILMENTS YOU CAN TREAT YOURSELF

In addition to chapters 1 to 10.

❧ **Abdominal pains:** relieved by pressure, lying face down or bent double; made worse by anger.

❧ **Facial neuralgia:** left-sided, comes and goes, made worse by movement or touch.

❧ **Sciatica:** often on the right, made worse by heat of the bed, improved by lying on painful side.

PERSONAL CHARACTERISTICS

YOU FEEL WORSE:
❧ Around 6 am or 4 to 5 pm.

YOU FEEL BETTER:
❧ For relieving pain by firm pressure.
❧ For drinking coffee.

MAIN USES
❧ For colicky pains and neuralgias.

Dulcamara

*S*olanum dulcamara, *commonly known as woody nightshade or bittersweet, is the source of this medicine.*

CONSTITUTIONAL AND PHYSICAL FEATURES
See pages 10–11

People who benefit from Dulcamara are often stout, rather opinionated and much involved in the problems of their own families. An outstanding physical feature is the onset or worsening of symptoms after exposure to cold, damp conditions. Dulcamara is an important medicine for the treatment of herpes infections and allergic conditions.

AILMENTS YOU CAN TREAT YOURSELF

In addition to those in chapters 1 to 10.

🐾 **Diarrhea:** aggravated by cold food and/or cold damp weather, especially in the summer when the days are hot and nights cold.

🐾 **Headaches:** caused by infected sinuses that are not discharging mucus.

🐾 **Rheumatism:** stiff joints or lower back pain, aggravated by cold, damp, getting wet.

🐾 **Skin:** flat smooth warts occurring on face and palms of hands.

🐾 **Urination:** frequent when cold.

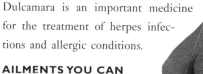

Ferrum phosphoricum

*I*ron phosphate is the *source of this medicine.*

CONSTITUTIONAL AND PHYSICAL FEATURES *See pages 10–11*

Thin, sensitive, rather nervous people respond well to Ferrum phosphoricum, but it will also help many other people in the early stages of an illness with a high fever, rapid pulse, weakness, drowsiness and unquenchable thirst. The face is flushed and mucus discharges from the nose may contain streaks of blood. Any headache may be relieved with cold compresses. The symptoms tend to be worse when perspiration does not occur.

AILMENTS YOU CAN TREAT YOURSELF

In addition to those in chapters 1 to 10.

🐾 **Frequent heavy periods:** with a bearing down sensation.

🐾 **Headache:** occurs during or just before a period, sometimes relieved by a nose bleed. Also headache that comes on from too much sun.

🐾 **Indigestion:** irregular vomiting of undigested food, with a poor appetite and aversion to meat and milk.

🐾 **Nosebleeds:** blood is bright red and oozes from the nose rather than gushes.

Gelsemium sempervirens

$\mathcal{G}$elsemium sempervirens *is also known as yellow jasmine, false jasmine, or Carolina jasmine.*

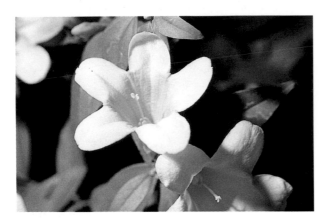

CONSTITUTIONAL AND PHYSICAL FEATURES *See pages 10–11*

Those best suited to Gelsemium sempervirens are often timid, reserved and unable to face up to a challenge, for example, stage fright. Symptoms include trembling, weakness, diarrhea, urgent urination and difficulty focusing or opening the eyes. The stress can lead to physical illness.

EMOTIONAL SYMPTOMS

There is a feeling of lassitude and dullness, and may feel unable or unwilling to think.

PERSONAL CHARACTERISTICS

YOU FEEL WORSE:
❧ In damp weather; before a thunderstorm.
❧ Anticipating a challenging event, e.g. public speaking or an interview.
❧ After a fright, bad news, any excitement.
❧ Around 10 am.
YOU FEEL BETTER:
❧ In the open air.
❧ After passing urine.
FOOD
❧ Not thirsty.
FEARS
❧ That heart will stop.

AILMENTS YOU CAN TREAT YOURSELF

In addition to those in chapters 1 to 10.
❧ **Head:** dull pain and heaviness in head, neck and shoulders, may be relieved by urination.
❧ **Trembling:** in extremities after slight exertion.
❧ **Heart:** fear that it will stop unless you move about.

MAIN USES
❧ For all types of weakness: mental, physical or emotional.

Graphites

$\mathcal{H}$*ahnemann made the first preparation of Graphites from the purest black-lead taken from a fine English pencil'. Chemically, black-lead consists of carbon but contains traces of iron. It is also known as graphite or plumbago.*

CONSTITUTIONAL AND PHYSICAL FEATURES
See pages 10–11

The Graphites 'type' is over-weight, has a fair complexion, is prone to various types of skin disease and abnormalities of the nails, and to constipation. A poor memory is common.

MAIN USES
❧ Skin conditions.

EMOTIONAL SYMPTOMS

May be difficult to think clearly or concentrate. Decisions may be difficult and music may cause sadness and even tears.

AILMENTS YOU CAN TREAT YOURSELF

In addition to those in chapters 1 to 10.
❧ **Conjunctivitis:** with a strong aversion to light.
❧ **Ears:** oozing cracks behind the ears; there is a discharge from the ear, but can hear better in noisy surroundings than in a quiet place.

PERSONAL CHARACTERISTICS

YOU FEEL WORSE:
❧ In the morning on waking.
❧ When discharges are suppressed, for example, a delayed period.
❧ In the cold but also in a hot bed.
YOU FEEL BETTER:
❧ After walking in the open air.
FOOD:
❧ A desire for chicken; bland food.
❧ An aversion to sweets, meat and fish.

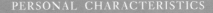

Hepar sulphuris calcareum

This medicine is derived from an impure form of calcium sulphide obtained, originally by Hahnemann, from heating finely powdered oyster shell with an equal weight of flowers of sulphur to a white heat for ten minutes. It is often known as Hepar sulph or just Hepar.

CONSTITUTIONAL AND PHYSICAL FEATURES *See pages 10–11*

Hepar sulphuris calcareum is most effective for people who are extraordinarily sensitive, both mentally and physically. It helps those who anger easily, cannot tolerate pain, being touched, or exposed to drafts or cold. They are impossible to please and extremely susceptible to infection.

EMOTIONAL SYMPTOMS

So sensitive to any outside influences that may be tempted not to venture out of the house. When something does happens, there is a tendency to react with anger, and illness causes depression, as you feel so awful, even when suffering from only minor complaints.

AILMENTS YOU CAN TREAT YOURSELF

In addition to those in chapters 1 to 10.

- **Facial neuralgia:** often right-sided, and very tender when it is touched.
- **Skin conditions:** tendency to an unhealthy skin, every cut suppurates and heals slowly; boils and abscesses are exquisitely tender to touch.
- **Sore throat:** the pain feels like a splinter in the throat and this may extend to the ear when swallowing; tonsils are swollen and discharge pus.

PERSONAL CHARACTERISTICS

YOU FEEL WORSE:
- If you become cold, are exposed to the cold, or touch something cold.
- In drafts, in cold dry winds.

YOU FEEL BETTER:
- For being covered up, especially your head.
- In damp weather.

FOOD
- A craving for fat, vinegar, pickles and spices.

FEARS
- Of hearing news of violent accidents.
- Of going to the dentist.
- Dream about fires.

MAIN USES
❧ Various infections.

Ignatia amara

MAIN USES
❧ After acute grief, and as a constitutional medicine.

This is made from the fruit of Ignatia amara, which acquired the name St Ignatius bean when the Spanish Jesuits introduced it to merchants in the 17th century. The plant is native to the Philippines and East Indies.

CONSTITUTIONAL AND PHYSICAL FEATURES *See pages 10–11*

Ignatia 'types' are romantic idealists who are apt to be dissatisfied with their circumstances in life, but they are also extremely sensitive to any disappointment. They find it difficult to talk about their emotional problems and become suspicious of offers of help, which often annoy them. Ignatia is often used for grief and/or romantic disappointment, and can help anyone who reacts to grief with rapidly changing moods, sighing and hysterical weeping

EMOTIONAL SYMPTOMS

May be dismayed by the fact that controlling emotions is more difficult than usual, and be embarrassed by weeping in front of other people. May long to get away and change things, and find the idea of travelling attractive. A fear of choking may result from feeling that there is an immovable lump in throat.

AILMENTS YOU CAN TREAT YOURSELF

In addition to those in chapters 1 to 10.

- **Cough:** in paroxysms without infection being present.
- **Diarrhea:** from fright or worrying about someone else; it may alternate with constipation.
- **Digestive problems:** stomach cramps that are made worse by external pressure; variable appetite; a sour taste in the mouth with excessive saliva and gas; a sinking feeling in the stomach helped by deep breathing; a tendency to bite the inner cheeks when chewing; morning sickness with a sinking sensation in the stomach that is improved by eating.
- **Headaches:** nervous headaches; with periods or after anger.

PERSONAL CHARACTERISTICS

YOU FEEL WORSE:
- After eating, especially sweets.
- Drinking coffee.
- For smoking or being in a smoky room.

YOU FEEL BETTER:
- For travelling or moving in the rain.

FOOD
- A craving for cheese.
- An aversion to fruit.

FEARS
- Of birds.
- Of being confined.

SLEEP
- May be excessive after grief.
- May dream of water.

Ipecacuanha

This medicine is made from the dried root of Psychotria (Cephaelis) ipecacuanha, which is native to Brazil. A syrup derived from this plant is still used in conventional medicine to induce vomiting in children after they have eaten a poisonous substance.

CONSTITUTIONAL AND PHYSICAL FEATURES *See pages 10–11*

Ipecacuanha can be used whenever there is nausea and/or vomiting either as the main condition or when associated with symptoms in other parts of the body, for example, with headaches, coughs or hemorrhage from the uterus (womb). The nausea is persistent even after vomiting, but the tongue remains clean and moist.

AILMENTS YOU CAN TREAT YOURSELF

In addition to those in chapters 1 to 10.

❧ **Heavy periods:** bright red bleeding that starts very suddenly and often comes in gushes: may also feel nauseous and faint.

MAIN USES
❧ Nausea and vomiting, asthma and hemorrhage.

PERSONAL CHARACTERISTICS

YOU FEEL WORSE:
❧ For warmth.
❧ For overeating, especially rich foods.
❧ For being sick.

YOU FEEL BETTER:
❧ In the open air.
❧ For rest and closing eyes.

FOOD
❧ An aversion to food.

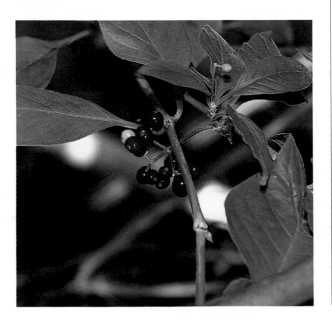

Kali bichromicum

The English name for the chemical used as the source of this medicine is Potassium bichromate.

CONSTITUTIONAL AND PHYSICAL FEATURES *See pages 10–11*

Although the Kali bichromicum 'type' is overweight, a conformist and prefers to keep a rigid routine, almost anyone who suffers from a thick gluey discharge from the nose, throat, or vagina will be helped by this medicine. Characteristically, those who respond best to Kali bichromicum feel generally weak and weary.

AILMENTS YOU CAN TREAT YOURSELF

In addition to those in chapters 1 to 10.

❧ **Arthritis:** that tends to wander from joint to joint. Sore heels that occur after walking. The joint pains come and go very suddenly.

❧ **Eye infection:** a sticky yellow discharge that occurs with excessive tears.

❧ **Indigestion:** symptoms come on soon after eating with heaviness in the stomach, distension with belching, aversion to water and intolerance of meat.

MAIN USES
❧ Thick gluey discharges, especially from the nose.
❧ Arthritis.

❧ **Sinusitis:** with thick, stringy, yellow discharge from the nose and/or throat. The pain is felt in a small area about the size of a finger tip.

❧ **Pain in the coccyx (tail bone):** aggravated by sitting, walking or touching it. It is relieved by urination or by sexual intercourse.

PERSONAL CHARACTERISTICS

YOU FEEL WORSE:
❧ In the cold and damp.
❧ Around 1 am.
❧ From drinking beer.

YOU FEEL BETTER:
❧ For moving about.

FOOD
❧ Potatoes and other starchy foods may be poorly digested.
❧ A craving for sweets.

Kali carbonicum

The potassium carbonate, from which this medicine is made, is derived from wood ash.

MAIN USES
⅋ Arthritis.
⅋ Catarrh and phlegm.
⅋ Asthma.
⅋ Indigestion.

CONSTITUTIONAL AND PHYSICAL FEATURES *See pages 10–11*

Kali carbonicum best suits those with a highly developed sense of right and wrong to which they adhere firmly. They may be obese, and prefer to dress conservatively. They are often stoical and tend not to consult a doctor until an illness is well advanced. Despite this, they can be discontented, weak, irritable and dislike change. Sudden noises can make them start.

AILMENTS YOU CAN TREAT YOURSELF
In addition to those in chapters 1 to 10.

Insomnia: sleeplessness caused by being unable to 'let go', or wakes up after four hours.

Nausea: from excitement, or from cold drinks when hot.

Puffiness of the eyelids: and face, due to allergies.

PERSONAL CHARACTERISTICS

YOU FEEL WORSE:
⅋ For any draft, however slight.
⅋ For cold weather.
⅋ Between 2 and 4 am.
⅋ For being touched.

YOU FEEL BETTER:
⅋ During the daytime.
⅋ For moving about.
⅋ In warm, wet weather.

FOOD
⅋ A craving for sweets.

FEARS
⅋ Of disease.
⅋ Of being alone.
⅋ Of the dark.
⅋ Fear is felt physically in the stomach.

Lachesis mutus

This medicine is made from the venom of Lachesis muta also known as the bushmaster or surucuccu snake, from South America. A homeopathic doctor, Constantine Hering, was accidentally poisoned by this venom in 1837 and a careful account of his symptoms was kept.

MAIN USES
⅋ As a constitutional medicine, but particularly for menopausal symptoms and depression.

CONSTITUTIONAL AND PHYSICAL FEATURES
See pages 10–11

Lachesis mutus best suits those people who might be described as 'intense'; they work hard and play hard. They overflow with ideas and are often very talkative, but they can fall into sullen, silent depression or anxiety. They are competitive and love passionately, but they are prone to jealousy and can become suspicious of their partners. They may become dependent on alcohol or drugs. Typically their complexion is puffy with a purplish tinge.

EMOTIONAL SYMPTOMS

A tendency to react to illness by feeling jealous, suspicious of others and/or more irritable than usual. Grief or disappointment following a love affair can initiate illnesses that will respond to Lachesis mutus. If depressed, this can be severe in the morning.

AILMENTS YOU CAN TREAT YOURSELF
In addition to those in chapters 1 to 10.

⅋ **Asthma:** often related to hayfever, or can follow jealousy or other strong emotions: feel suffocated, need to loosen clothes and open the window: made worse by a hot room, lying down, during the night or on waking.

⅋ **Back pain and sciatica:** back pain radiating to the hips and legs; sciatica during pregnancy.

⅋ **Facial neuralgia:** burning left-sided pain, which may extend to head.

PERSONAL CHARACTERISTICS

YOU FEEL WORSE:
⅋ For any constriction or pressure, e.g. tight clothing.
⅋ After sleep.
⅋ For heat – a warm bath or hot drink.
⅋ In the spring.

YOU FEEL BETTER:
⅋ At the start of a discharge, e.g. a period or the bursting of a carbuncle.
⅋ In the open air.

FOOD
⅋ A craving for alcohol, starchy food and cold drinks.

FEARS
⅋ Of snakes.
⅋ Of being poisoned.

SLEEP
⅋ Usually on the right side.
⅋ May be disturbed by sudden sensation of suffocation.
⅋ Nightmares.

Lilium tigrinum

Also known as the tiger lily, this plant is native to China and Japan. The medicine is prepared from the stalk, leaves and flowers.

CONSTITUTIONAL AND PHYSICAL FEATURES *See pages 10–11*

Women who need Lilium tigrinum often have a deep inner conflict about their strong desire for sexual fulfilment and the feeling that this is wrong. If they suppress their sexual energy they can become frantic and fear insanity. This state can alternate with great kindness and concern for others. These women tend to feel very hurried and can, as a result of this, become very unproductive.

> MAIN USES
> ❦ For women.

EMOTIONAL SYMPTOMS:

You are likely to react to your inner conflicts by anger and irritability. You may take offence easily and refuse any sympathy from people.

AILMENTS YOU CAN TREAT YOURSELF

In addition to those in chapters 1 to 10.

❦ **Bowel problems:** constant desire to move the bowels but unable to do so. Urgent evacuation in the early morning.

❦ **Period problems:** great irritability premenstrually. Bearing down sensation, as if pelvic organs will drop out, aggravated during a period. Constant desire to urinate.

❦ **Restless legs:** due to constant aching.

❦ **Rheumatism:** pains in ankles, right arm and hip. Burning feet. Unable to walk on rough ground.

PERSONAL CHARACTERISTICS

YOU FEEL WORSE:
❦ For being warm.
❦ Standing up (because of a feeling that the pelvic organs will drop down).
❦ After sexual intercourse.

YOU FEEL BETTER:
❦ In the open air.
❦ For being busy.

FOOD
❦ A craving for meat.

FEARS
❦ Of insanity.
❦ Of heart disease.
❦ 'That something bad will happen.'

Lycopodium clavatum

Lycopodium clavatum is a moss-like plant. Before Hahnemann potentized its spores it was thought to be without medicinal action, and was used by pharmacists to prevent pills sticking to each other. Common names for the plant include wolf's claws and club moss.

> MAIN USES
> ❦ As a constitutional medicine, for digestive disorders.

CONSTITUTIONAL AND PHYSICAL FEATURES
See pages 10–11

Lycopodium clavatum is used for many illnesses, both acute and chronic, and can help many different people. However, it is particularly useful for shy, intellectual types, who are not physically strong. They often lack self-confidence and dread appearing before an audience but, when they do, they perform well. They do not want company but like to know there is someone nearby. They sometimes find difficulty in making a long-term commitment, such as marriage. Physically they tend to look anxious, with a frown above the nose, and the skin may be a sallow color, old-looking with prematurely grey hair.

EMOTIONAL SYMPTOMS

Tendency to be anxious about things, particularly about the outcome of illness, possibly forgetful, sometimes sentimental, and may weep on being thanked.

AILMENTS YOU CAN TREAT YOURSELF

In addition to those in chapters 1 to 10.

❦ **Headache:** usually right-sided, may be neuralgic, worst between 4 and 8 pm, aggravated by heat in bed and if not eating regularly.

❦ **Joints and muscles:** burning pain between shoulder blades.

PERSONAL CHARACTERISTICS

YOU FEEL WORSE:
❦ In late afternoon between 4 and 8 pm.
❦ On waking in the morning.
❦ If you miss a meal.
❦ If you get chilled.
❦ If clothes are tight

YOU FEEL BETTER:
❦ In the open air even if not very warm.
❦ For moving about after warm meals.

FOOD
❦ A craving for sweets.
❦ Indigestion from starchy food, cabbage and beans.
❦ An aversion to cold drinks.
❦ May feel full after only a few mouthfuls despite being very hungry before eating.

FEARS
❦ Of being alone, especially at night.
❦ Of ghosts.
❦ Of serious illness.
❦ Of public speaking.

SLEEP
❦ Is often unrefreshing.
❦ Have to sleep on the right side and may wake with hunger.

Mercurius solubilis

This medicine is prepared from quicksilver. Of all the homeopathic medicines based on mercury this is the one most frequently used, and you may find that it is simply called Mercurius.

CONSTITUTIONAL AND PHYSICAL FEATURES *See pages 10–11*

Like mercury in a thermometer, the people most likely to be helped by Mercurius solubilis are very sensitive to any change in temperature. They are reserved and mistrustful, but underneath a calm exterior they can have strong feelings and are prone to sudden impulses. They can have many fears, and sometimes develop a sense of being hurried.

AILMENTS YOU CAN TREAT YOURSELF

In addition to those in chapters 1 to 10.

❦ **Arthritis:** swelling of joints, a cold sensation.

PERSONAL CHARACTERISTICS

YOU FEEL WORSE:
- ❦ At night.
- ❦ For both heat and cold.
- ❦ After sweating.
- ❦ In damp weather.

YOU FEEL BETTER:
- ❦ In moderate temperatures.

FOOD
- ❦ A craving for bread and butter.
- ❦ An aversion to sweets.

FEARS
- ❦ Of disease and death.
- ❦ Of darkness.
- ❦ Of poverty.

SLEEP
- ❦ There is tremor in the extremities, especially in the hands.
- ❦ Night sweats.

MAIN USES
- ❦ Colds.
- ❦ Tonsillitis.
- ❦ Digestive upsets.

Natrum muriaticum

The English name for this medicine is sodium chloride, but it is much better known as common salt.

CONSTITUTIONAL AND PHYSICAL FEATURES
See pages 10–11

Natrum muriaticum is most frequently used for illness caused through grief, fright or anger, particularly when these strong emotions have been suppressed and not fully resolved. People most likely to benefit are responsible and perfectionists, but highly sensitive and open to being deeply hurt by life's experiences. They are often unable to talk about their feelings although they may brood over past griefs. Alternatively their pain gradually becomes almost forgotten, but sadness wells up when something occurs to remind them of the event.

MAIN USES
- ❦ As a constitutional medicine.

EMOTIONAL SYMPTOMS

May wish to be left alone when ill and reject anyone who attempts consolation. May also be very sensitive to noise, including music, and intolerant of bright light. Drowning pain in alcohol may sometimes be a very tempting solution.

AILMENTS YOU CAN TREAT YOURSELF
In addition to those in chapters 1 to 10.

❦ **Back pain:** especially in the lower back, relieved by lying against something firm.

❦ **Headache:** often before or after a period, or caused by grief. It may feel like hammers in the head and often occurs around 10 am or from sunrise to sunset: made worse by light, sun or noise, but improved by lying in the dark and using some cold compresses.

❦ **Head colds:** these often start with sneezing and clear discharge from the nose. Eyes may feel bruised and heavy, and are prone to water freely especially in the wind.

PERSONAL CHARACTERISTICS

YOU FEEL WORSE:
- ❦ In hot sun.
- ❦ At the seaside.
- ❦ Around 10 am (may need to eat).

YOU FEEL BETTER:
- ❦ When alone.

FOOD
- ❦ A desire for salt, sour food and cold drinks.
- ❦ An aversion to fat, rich and slimy foods.

FEARS
- ❦ Of burglars.
- ❦ Of confined spaces.
- ❦ Of germs.

Nitricum acidum

*N*itricum acidum is a strong, corrosive acid that was once known as aqua fortis, and was introduced to homeopathy by Hahnemann himself.

CONSTITUTIONAL AND PHYSICAL FEATURES *See pages 10–11*

People who are constitutionally suited to Nitricum acidum are often dark complexioned, have a hopeless despair about their illness and an overwhelming fear of death. They tend to be vindictive, headstrong and irritable, especially first thing in the morning. However, Nitricum acidum is used most frequently for people without this gloomy personality but whose illness matches the physical feature described for this medicine throughout this book. They may experience offensive sweat, urine or feces.

PERSONAL CHARACTERISTICS

YOU FEEL WORSE:
- When cold.
- In the evening.

YOU FEEL BETTER:
- When in a vehicle.

FOOD
- A strong craving for fat and salt.
- Indigestion from milk.
- Always hungry.

FEARS
- Of cancer, AIDS and death.
- Of poverty.

SLEEP
- Wake at 2 am.

MAIN USES
- Conditions that affect areas where the skin and the mucous membranes (soft pink lining of the mouth, eyelids etc.) meet, for example, around the mouth, anus etc.
- It is also a constitutional medicine.

AILMENTS YOU CAN TREAT YOURSELF

In addition to those in chapters 1 to 10.

- **Anal fissure (split) and hemorrhoids:** the rectum and anus feel torn, may bleed and hurt violently for hours after passing some stool.
- **Catarrh:** green crusts in the nose each morning, or yellow offensive nasal discharge. Nose may also be sore and bleeding.
- **Warts:** Nitricum acidum can be used to treat warts affecting those parts of the body where the skin and mucous membranes meet, for example, around the anus, in the genital area around the vulva, on the face around the lips (see also page 16). The warts may feel sore and be prone to bleeding. There may also be some sore cracks at the corners of the mouth (see also page 108).

Nux vomica

*T*his is prepared from Strychnos nux vomica *which is commonly called the poison nut plant. As the botanical name suggests, the plant contains strychnine.*

CONSTITUTIONAL AND PHYSICAL FEATURES *See pages 10–11*

Nux vomica 'types' are impatient, ambitious workaholics with a need to be extremely clean and tidy. They tend to be very competitive both at work and recreation, and collapse from overwork. However, Nux vomica is eminently suitable for the stresses of overwork and modern living, and many people will benefit from it.

EMOTIONAL SYMPTOMS

May be prone to anger when things go wrong and either break things or weep. However, also very sensitive to criticism, other people, noise, light, odors etc. Tend to drink too much coffee or alcohol, or use drugs in order to cope.

AILMENTS YOU CAN TREAT YOURSELF

In addition to those in chapters 1 to 10.

- **Asthma:** aggravated by exertion, around 3 to 4 am or in the morning, in the cold.
- **Headaches:** may be associated with too much food or alcohol, after being too long in the sun or around the time of your periods. Pain may be aggravated by noise, light, having to think or by just being annoyed.
- **Lumbago:** feeling as if back is broken: need to sit up in bed to turn over.
- **Sleep problems:** drowsy after eating and in early evening: wakeful between 3 and 4 am in the morning: although may get back to sleep, could still wake in the morning feeling unrefreshed.

PERSONAL CHARACTERISTICS

YOU FEEL WORSE:
- In cold weather, especially in a cold dry wind.
- In a draft.
- After eating.

YOU FEEL BETTER:
- After uninterrupted sleep or catnap.
- In damp weather.

FOOD
- A desire for stimulants, fat and spicy food.

FEARS
- Of failure.
- Of marriage.
- Of humiliation.
- Of darkness.

MAIN USES
- As a constitutional medicine, most frequently for digestive disorders.

Phosphoricum acidum

Hahnemann used bones and sulphuric acid to prepare this medicine, but today commercial phosphoric acid is used.

CONSTITUTIONAL AND PHYSICAL FEATURES *See pages 10–11*

Phosphoricum acidum is needed for people who are in a state of collapse, in particular after grief, but also after debilitating illness, and occasionally after drug abuse or alcoholism.

EMOTIONAL SYMPTOMS

May feel overwhelmed by this condition, emotionally flat and indifferent, and feel fatigued and drained. May also find that memory is impaired and that brain is working very slowly.

AILMENTS YOU CAN TREAT YOURSELF

In addition to those in chapters 1 to 10.

❧ **Arthritis and cramps:** weakness of the limbs, cramps in the arms.

❧ **Cough and shortage of breath:** weakness in chest from coughing and talking.

❧ **Headache:** four types – pressure on top of the head, pain as if temples being pressed together, after sexual intercourse, from eyestrain.

❧ **Indigestion:** after sour food and drink.

❧ **Mouth conditions:** dry, cracked lips and bleeding gums; a swollen, dry tongue that may be accidentally bitten at night when asleep.

❧ **Urinary conditions:** frequent, profuse urination especially at night.

PERSONAL CHARACTERISTICS

YOU FEEL WORSE:
❧ From exertion, including being talked to.
❧ After sexual intercourse.

YOU FEEL BETTER:
❧ After sleep.
❧ Being warm.

FOOD
❧ A craving for fruit and fruit juices.

MAIN USES
❧ For collapse and grief.

Phosphorus

Phosphorus is a common element in both plants and animals, and bone ash is the source for the homeopathic medicine.

CONSTITUTIONAL AND PHYSICAL FEATURES
See pages 10–11

When well, people who are Phosphorus 'types' can best be described as 'the life and soul of the party'. They show enormous enthusiasm for life and great sympathy for the plight of others, even complete strangers. However, they also depend on the support of other people, and are prone to many fears particularly when they are alone. They tend to take up a cause with vigor and then drop it suddenly. They spend freely and borrow money with little thought about repayment of their debts. Physically they are often tall and thin, sometimes with auburn hair, and have limited stamina. Usually they are chilly and feel the cold but are sometimes intolerant of heat.

MAIN USES
❧ As a constitutional medicine, particularly for chest and digestive disorders, and bleeding.

EMOTIONAL SYMPTOMS

When ill, and especially if alone, there may be fears that can become insurmountable and cause a lapse into depression. This could lead to a feeling of hopelessness and a tendency to brood about this condition. Easily startled and may also have out-of-body experiences.

AILMENTS YOU CAN TREAT YOURSELF

In addition to those in chapters 1 to 10.

❧ **Angina:** may be used with conventional medicine if angina is developed from stress, it is worse lying on your left side.

❧ **Cough:** a hard, dry persistent hacking cough, sometimes with burning chest pain, made worse by cold air, exertion, talking and laughing, lying on the left side.

❧ **Hemorrhage:** nose bleeds, excessive bleeding after tooth extraction, bleeding from the anus.

PERSONAL CHARACTERISTICS

YOU FEEL WORSE:
❧ If you do not eat regularly or try to fast.
❧ Lying on left side.
❧ During twilight.
❧ For putting hands in cold water.

YOU FEEL BETTER:
❧ After eating and from cold drinks.
❧ For being caressed and after massage.
❧ After sleep.

FOOD:
❧ A craving for chocolate, salt, ice cream and cold food.
❧ A desire for spicy food, rice, milk and wine
❧ An aversion to sweets and warm food.

FEARS:
❧ Of thunderstorms.
❧ 'That something bad will happen.'
❧ Of being alone or in the dark.
❧ Of death and life-threatening disease.

Psorinum

This medicine is derived from the contents of an infected skin lesion resulting from the scabies mite burrowing into the skin. Once it is prepared homeopathically it is, of course, no longer capable of causing any further infection.

CONSTITUTIONAL AND PHYSICAL FEATURES *See pages 10–11*

Psorinum suits people who are pessimistic and feel the cold weather very keenly. They accept poverty and disappointment and settle for less than they could achieve, but this brings depression and isolation. The skin looks as if it is unwashed even after washing. People who need Psoriunum are prone to recurrent infections. Discharges, for example, from the nose, ears or skin, often smell offensive.

MAIN USES
❧ Most systems in the body, but particularly the skin.

PERSONAL CHARACTERISTICS

YOU FEEL WORSE:
❧ In cold weather, open air, or drafts.
❧ At night.

YOU FEEL BETTER:
❧ When warm, may need warm clothing, even in summer heat.

FOOD
❧ There is an aversion to coffee.
❧ Can get hungry at night.

FEARS
❧ Of poverty.
❧ Of the future.
❧ Of failure.
❧ Of serious health problems.

EMOTIONAL SYMPTOMS

Depression and anxiety about the future are compounded by the fear of never being well again and/or have been abandoned. Anxiety is worse at night.

AILMENTS YOU CAN TREAT YOURSELF

In addition to those in chapters 1 to 10.

❧ **Chest complaints:** cough, bronchitis or asthma, exhausted, shortage of breath relieved by lying flat with arms stretched out to the sides.

❧ **Eczema:** tremendous itching, which is worse at night, aggravated by heat of bed; a compulsion to scratch until it bleeds.

Pulsatilla

Pulsatilla pratensis subsp. nigricans, also known as the wind-flower, meadow anemone or pasque flower, grows on a chalky soil. The entire plant is used in the preparation of the medicine.

CONSTITUTIONAL AND PHYSICAL FEATURES
See pages 10–11

Pulsatilla 'types' are highly emotional, timid, irresolute women who cry easily and need sympathy and frequent caresses. Physically they are blue-eyed, fair-haired and pale. However, there are many women who will be helped by Pulsatilla at times when their circumstances cause them to develop some of the Pulsatilla 'type' characteristics. It can also help when their symptoms are caused by hormonal changes.

EMOTIONAL SYMPTOMS

May feel in need of support from friends and relatives and have a tendency to cry a lot. Emotions may be blown in every direction. May change mind after every piece of differing advice, but can also be very stubborn when own sense of security is threatened. The emotional symptoms are worsened by being confined in a hot, closed room, premenstrually, and in the evening.

AILMENTS YOU CAN TREAT YOURSELF

In addition to those in chapters 1 to 10.

❧ **Asthma:** often allergic, with shortage of breath.

❧ **Arthritis:** joint pains go from joint to joint, are worse on first moving and relieved by bathing.

❧ **Digestive conditions:** distension and pain after eating, especially rich, fatty foods. Alternating diarrhea and constipation occurs.

MAIN USES
❧ As a constitutional medicine, particularly during pregnancy.
❧ For hormonal problems in women and for circulatory disorders.

PERSONAL CHARACTERISTICS

YOU FEEL WORSE:
❧ At twilight and in the evening.
❧ After rich or fatty food (even though may desire these).
❧ If a period is late.
❧ When overheated or in the sun.
❧ After a sudden soaking.

YOU FEEL BETTER:
❧ For consolation and reassurance.
❧ When walking gently in the open air.

FOOD
❧ A craving for butter and cream.
❧ A desire for ice cream, cheese and cold food.
❧ An aversion to fat and pork.
❧ Not thirsty even when feverish.

FEARS
❧ Of high places.
❧ Of confined spaces.
❧ Of going mad.

SLEEP
❧ Often on the back with hands above the head.

Rhus toxicodendron

*C*ommonly known as poison ivy, this plant is native to North America and can cause a skin rash in sensitive people unwise enough to walk near it. When prepared homeopathically it can cure rashes that look similar to those it causes.

> **MAIN USES**
> ❧ For rheumatic conditions, but it also has some constitutional features.

CONSTITUTIONAL AND PHYSICAL FEATURES *See pages 10–11*

Those most likely to benefit from Rhus toxicodendron, when it is used constitutionally, are lively and cheerful when well, but when ill tend to become restless, agitated, depressed and sometimes superstitious. The tip of the tongue may be very red. However, Rhus toxicodendron is most frequently used to relieve rheumatic conditions in a wide variety of people, when there is progressive stiffness and pain that is made worse by damp, cold weather, before storms, on first moving in the morning and after overexertion. Typically the symptoms are better in warm, dry weather, after a warm bath and when moving about.

AILMENTS YOU CAN TREAT YOURSELF

In addition to those in chapters 1 to 10.

❧ **Influenza:** when the pain forces movement to a more comfortable position, but still do not feel comfortable for long and have to move again. Fever may come on rapidly around 10 pm.

❧ **Neck pain and stiffness:** caused or made worse by an injury or overuse. Improved by stretching the neck and moving the head about, and from warmth, especially a hot shower.

PERSONAL CHARACTERISTICS

YOU FEEL WORSE:
❧ In cold, damp, cloudy or foggy weather.
❧ In the autumn.
❧ In the evening, especially after having done too much.

YOU FEEL BETTER:
❧ For moving about; may find it impossible to keep still.
❧ After a massage.
❧ After a warm bath.

FOOD
❧ A craving for cold milk.

FEAR
❧ When thinking of sad things.

Sabina

*T*he medicinal properties of Juniperus sabina, *from which Sabina is made, were first recognized by the physicians of ancient Greece. The common name for the plant is savine.*

CONSTITUTIONAL AND PHYSICAL FEATURES *See pages 10–11*

Sabina best suits women who are intolerant of hot weather and do not feel the cold. They may be easily startled by sudden noise and intolerant of small noises. A marked feature of Sabina is its use in hemorrhagic conditions of all types , and it is most frequently used for heavy periods. It also relieves the pain of joints affected by arthritis and gout, and is one of the few medicines that are indicated when the joint symptoms are worse in hot weather or warm rooms

PERSONAL CHARACTERISTICS

YOU FEEL WORSE:
❧ During the night.
❧ In heat, being warm after exertion.
❧ In foggy weather.

YOU FEEL BETTER:
❧ In the open air.
❧ When cool.

FOOD
❧ A desire for lemons and salt.

> **MAIN USES**
> ❧ Conditions affecting the uterus (womb).

AILMENTS YOU CAN TREAT YOURSELF

In addition to those in chapters 1 to 10.

❧ **Back pain:** lower back pain either extending to the pubic bones or from them to the back.

❧ **Nose:** a tendency to nose bleeds, especially during a heavy period, or when a period is late.

❧ **Arthritis and gout:** red, swollen, tender joints. Pain is aggravated by heat, by moving about, by the joint being touched. Cool, open air brings relief.

Sanguinaria canadensis

Commonly known as blood root, Sanguinaria canadensis is a native of deciduous woods in North America and was used as a domestic medicine for winter colds before it was incorporated into homeopathic practice.

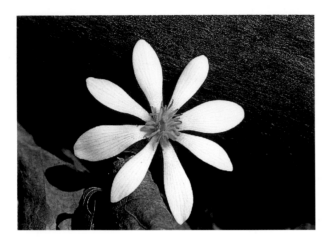

CONSTITUTIONAL AND PHYSICAL FEATURES *See pages 10–11*

Sanguinaria is of most use for right-sided conditions, particularly those that recur every seven days, for example, migraines that occur on weekends.

AILMENTS YOU CAN TREAT YOURSELF

In addition to those in chapters 1 to 10.

✐ **Asthma:** caused by grass or flower pollens, often associated with digestive upset.

✐ **Cough:** can cause vomiting but can also be relieved by vomiting; aggravated by lying down.

✐ **Hayfever:** a watery discharge occurs.

✐ **Shoulder pain:** usually on the right side and is aggravated by turning over in bed, trying to raise the arm, or by lying on the affected side.

MAIN USES
✵ Allergies.
✵ Migraines.
✵ Joint conditions.
✵ Menopausal flushes.

PERSONAL CHARACTERISTICS

YOU ARE WORSE:
✐ **When moving about.**
✐ **For being touched.**

YOU ARE BETTER:
✐ **For sleep.**

FOOD
✐ **A craving for spicy food.**
✐ **An aversion to butter.**

Sepia

Sepia officinalis is the common cuttlefish and the liquid found in its ink sac is the source of this medicine. It was introduced to homeopathy by Hahnemann, who treated an artist whose illness resulted from using cuttlefish ink in his work.

MAIN USES
✵ As a constitutional medicine for women.

CONSTITUTIONAL AND PHYSICAL FEATURES
See pages 10–11

Sepia is most likely to help women who are exhausted. They rely on their sense of duty to keep going because their reserves of energy are drained by the need to love and care for their families. Their exhaustion makes them feel stupid and dull. The demands of the family make them angry and they may lash out, but this creates remorse which adds to their desperation. By contrast, if they make the effort to go to a party or take vigorous exercise they feel truly better. Physically, they are often tall, thin and flat chested, but many plump women have also been helped by Sepia. A brownish-yellow saddle-shaped discoloration may be present on the nose and cheeks. Chronic headaches, backache, constipation, excessive perspiration all contribute to a 'dragged-down' feeling that is typical of those needing Sepia. It is a medicine that is often needed by women today, as they juggle with the demands of combining a career with raising a family.

EMOTIONAL SYMPTOMS

May feel pathetic, worn out and weepy, reluctant to be in company yet not truly happy on own. Vigorous exercise, especially dancing or aerobics, or watching a thunderstorm may lead to feeling better. May suffer from a loss of sexual desire and dislike being touched sexually. Even if feeling overworked, will still refuse offers of help.

AILMENTS YOU CAN TREAT YOURSELF

In addition to those in chapters 1 to 10.

✐ **Headaches:** often left-sided, can be aggravated by fasting, during a period or during the menopause.

PERSONAL CHARACTERISTICS

YOU FEEL WORSE:
✐ **Before and during a period.**
✐ **During the afternoon hours.**
✐ **At the seaside.**
✐ **After diarrhea.**

YOU FEEL BETTER:
✐ **After vigorous exercise.**

FOOD
✐ **A craving for sweets, vinegar, sour foods, plus an aversion to fat.**

FEARS
✐ **Of ghosts.**
✐ **Of poverty.**

Silicea

This medicine is prepared from silicon dioxide which occurs naturally in flint, quartz, sandstone and other minerals.

CONSTITUTIONAL AND PHYSICAL FEATURES *See pages 10–11*

People needing Silicea are often refined, delicate and sensitive, especially to noise, but they lack 'grit'. Emotionally, this leads to a poorly developed sense of self-esteem. Physically, they not only lack stamina but are prone to infections of the respiratory system, the skin, the mouth and the rectum. The bones, nails or teeth can be weak and defective.

EMOTIONAL SYMPTOMS

May feel unable to cope with what needs to be done and because of doubts about own ability there may also be a tendency to compensate by concentrating on details. Not only does this annoy other people, but leads to great anxiety about getting things right and may find making decisions very difficult.

> ### MAIN USES
> ❧ Conditions in which stamina is low.

AILMENTS YOU CAN TREAT YOURSELF

In addition to those in chapters 1 to 10.

❧ **Headaches:** which often begin at the back of head and extend to forehead or right side of the head. They can be made worse from cold, thinking, during a period or after uncovering head. These headaches can be relieved by closing eyes, lying down in the dark, or from warmth especially from wrapping head.

❧ **Abscesses:** wherever they occur in the body: dental, breast, vulval (Bartholin's cyst), rectal.

> ### PERSONAL CHARACTERISTICS
>
> *YOU FEEL WORSE:*
> ❧ In cold weather, or in cold drafts.
> ❧ When uncovered: may want a hat even in warm weather.
>
> *YOU FEEL BETTER:*
> ❧ In warm damp weather.
>
> *FOOD*
> ❧ A desire for ice cream, sweets and eggs.
> ❧ An aversion to fat, meat, cooked or warm food.
>
> *FEARS:*
> ❧ Stage fright.
> ❧ Of pointed objects such as pins.

Staphysagria

Medicine derived from Delphinium staphisagria was used at the time of Hippocrates. The homeopathic medicine is prepared from the seeds of the plant commonly known as stavesacre or palmated larkspur.

CONSTITUTIONAL AND PHYSICAL FEATURES *See pages 10–11*

People who need Staphysagria find confrontation difficult and suppress their feelings. Frequently they do not feel anger in the same way that most people would: they appear outwardly very sweet-natured although they may confess to feelings of guilt or shame. Eventually they give way to outbursts of anger in which they may throw things. Their inner thoughts and fantasies are often of a sexual nature.

EMOTIONAL SYMPTOMS

May have suffered many griefs in the past, but not felt able, for a variety of reasons, to express feelings. May weep easily and lack self-confidence.

AILMENTS YOU CAN TREAT YOURSELF

In addition to those in chapters 1 to 10.

❧ **Insomnia:** unable to sleep at night, but drowsy feelings in the daytime.

> ### MAIN USES
> ❧ Ailments resulting from suppressed anger or grief.

❧ **Psoriasis:** after grief or suppression of strong emotions.

> ### PERSONAL CHARACTERISTICS
>
> *YOU FEEL WORSE:*
> ❧ After a daytime nap.
> ❧ When emotions are aroused.
>
> *YOU FEEL BETTER*
> ❧ For warmth.
>
> *FOOD*
> ❧ A desire for sweets and bread.
>
> *FEARS*
> ❧ Of high places.
> ❧ Of anger.

Sulphur

he word 'sulphur' is Latin for burning stone which was corrupted into the English 'brimstone'. Sulphur has been used for religious and purification purposes since prehistoric times. The homeopathic medicine is prepared from flowers of sulphur.

PERSONAL CHARACTERISTICS

YOU FEEL WORSE:
❧ If too warm, especially in bed.
❧ In winter and when the weather is cloudy.
❧ For bathing.

YOU FEEL BETTER:
❧ When lying down.

FOOD
❧ A craving for sweets, ice cream, fatty food, spices, alcohol and ice-cold drinks.
❧ An aversion to eggs.
❧ May crave chocolate and sweet things before periods.

FEAR
❧ Of high places.
❧ Of disease.
❧ Of failure.

SLEEP
❧ Prefer to lie on left side.
❧ May get nightmares if lie on back.

CONSTITUTIONAL AND PHYSICAL FEATURES
See pages 10–11

Sulphur is said to be needed by men more frequently than by women, but there are many women who have benefited from this medicine. On the whole, people who need Sulphur have intellectual gifts which they exercise either as detached thinkers or as practical and competent doers. Most of them are self-confident but they tend to be self-absorbed and quick to find fault. They cannot stand for long, as this can cause symptoms, for example, pain or diarrhea; and are typically very hungry at 11 am. Physically, they may be thin with round shoulders or can tend to obesity.

EMOTIONAL SYMPTOMS

May experience anxiety about health, and have fears on behalf of the family. A bad smell may cause feelings of disgust, as can certain objects or people.

AILMENTS YOU CAN TREAT YOURSELF

In addition to those in chapters 1 to 10.
❧ **Arthritis:** often affects left shoulder and is relieved by the application of cold compresses.
❧ **Conjunctivitis and inflammation of the eyelids:** eyes are red in the day and itch at night. Eyes may feel as if they are burning, and difficult to open in the morning.
❧ **Diarrhea:** or soft stool first thing in the morning, and may be worse after alcohol.

Thuja occidentalis

huja occidentalis has been called the white cedar, or tree of life (Arbor vitae). It is native to North America and the fresh green twigs were first used in homeopathy by Hahnemann.

CONSTITUTIONAL AND PHYSICAL FEATURES *See pages 10–11*

Thuja (pronounced thoo-ya) occidentalis helps people

who feel depressed and lack confidence. Sometimes they have strange fixed ideas about their bodies, believing them to be made of glass and breakable, or that there is something live inside them. Often there is a history of neglect or abuse in childhood, and their greatest wish is to be acceptable and accepted. However, many people who do not experience these feelings can be helped by Thuja occidentalis.

EMOTIONAL SYMPTOMS

May fear being very frank about inner thoughts and feelings.

AILMENTS YOU CAN TREAT YOURSELF

In addition to those in chapters 1 to 10.
❧ **Asthma:** that is worse in damp weather.
❧ **Headache:** feels like a nail being driven into your head.

PERSONAL CHARACTERISTICS

YOU FEEL WORSE:
❧ When the weather is cold and/or damp.
❧ Around 3 am and 3 pm.

YOU FEEL BETTER:
❧ After sweating.
❧ Following a massage.

FOOD:
❧ A desire for sweets.
❧ May crave or have an aversion to onions, garlic or tea.
❧ Onions may be upsetting.

FEARS
❧ Of not being liked.

SLEEP
❧ Prefer the left side, and may dream of falling.
❧ May wake around 3 to 4 am.

Veratrum album

The homeopathic medicine is prepared from the roots of this plant, commonly known as white false hellebore.

MAIN USES
❧ Ailments associated with cold sweats, but it also has some constitutional features.

CONSTITUTIONAL AND PHYSICAL FEATURES *See pages 10–11*
Veratrum album can be used by homeopaths to treat psychiatric disorders in which there is mental overstimulation, mood changes and dissociation from reality. The uses described in this book are confined to physical indications.

AILMENTS YOU CAN TREAT YOURSELF
In addition to those in chapters 1 to 10.

❧ **Gastroenteritis:** profuse vomiting and diarrhea usually with a cold sweat.

❧ **Extremities:** extreme coldness and pallor is felt, especially from various activities, such as using vibrating machinery, playing the piano or typing (Raynaud's syndrome).

❧ **Vertigo:** with vomiting and cold sweat.

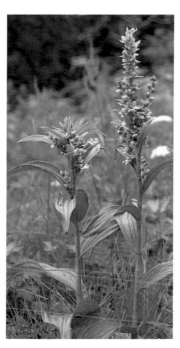

PERSONAL CHARACTERISTICS

YOU FEEL WORSE:
❧ In cold temperatures.
❧ At night.
YOU FEEL BETTER:
❧ When warm.
❧ When walking about.
FOOD
❧ A craving for sour food and fruit, lemons, salt, and ice.
❧ A great thirst, especially for cold drinks.

Zincum metallicum

Metallic zinc was probably first isolated in India in the 13th century, and it was introduced to homeopathy by Hahnemann. Its main use in conventional medicine has been as a constituent of ointments.

CONSTITUTIONAL AND PHYSICAL FEATURES *See pages 10–11*
Zincum metallicum best suits those who are physically and mentally broken down. They appear lethargic and stupid, repeating everything that is said to them. However, moods can vary greatly between depression and elation. They sometimes complain constantly and seem unable to be satisfied. They are prone to develop twitching and/or trembling when chronically ill.

EMOTIONAL SYMPTOMS
May find that speech is affected because concentration is difficult and may be particularly averse to conversation and any other source of noise. Symptoms may improve once a discharge, especially period, starts or when a rash appears. On becoming angry or doing too much, there is a tendency to become exhausted.

AILMENTS YOU CAN TREAT YOURSELF
In addition to those in chapters 1 to 10.

❧ **Chilblains:** painful, but are better when rubbed.

❧ **Headache:** after wine, even a very small amount; the condition is aggravated in the open air.

❧ **Restless legs:** feet and legs are constantly moving when asleep, which as a result may be disturbed by jerks and kicks.

MAIN USES
❧ Conditions involving the nervous system.

PERSONAL CHARACTERISTICS

YOU FEEL WORSE:
❧ After wine or other alcoholic drinks.
❧ In the cold or after cold bathing.
YOU FEEL BETTER:
❧ While eating.
❧ For moving around.
❧ When a period starts or a rash erupts.
FOOD
❧ An aversion to fish or sweets.
❧ Feel very hungry around 11 am.

Glossary

AGGRAVATION

Symptoms are sometimes made worse after a homeopathic medicine has been taken and this is known as an aggravation. If you experience an aggravation consult pages 10–11.

CONSTITUTIONAL TREATMENT

This is based on the whole personality of the patient, including inherited predisposition, experiences in life, emotional and intellectual attributes, and physical reactions to the environment. Occasionally physique, skin and hair colouring etc. are important. A prescription that takes these features into account is sometimes known as a constitutional medicine.

MATERIA MEDICA

In homeopathy the term *materia medica* is used to describe the collection of the symptoms that a particular medicine can be used to relieve.

METABOLISM

The process of chemical change that is continually taking place in the body is known as metabolism. Complex substances, such as proteins, are made from simpler substances and other complex substances are broken down into simpler ones, usually with the release of energy.

MOTHER TINCTURE

The mother tincture is the concentrated medicine from which the potencies are made.

POTENCY

A potency is made when a very small amount of mother tincture is systematically diluted in a mixture of water and alcohol, and vigorously shaken between each dilution (see page 10).

PROVINGS

Samuel Hahnemann recorded the symptoms that homeopathic medicines could both cause and cure (see page 10) by giving the medicines to healthy people. He called these symptoms 'provings', and they can occasionally occur after you have taken a homeopathic medicine for an illness (see pages 10–11).

SYMPTOM MEDICINE

A symptom medicine is a prescription that depends on the symptoms that the patient is experiencing. The symptoms may be directly related to the illness, such as a painful knee in arthritis, or more general, such as a thirst for cold drinks. The chance of a successful outcome is increased when as many features as possible match those described for the medicine.

Bibliography

A BRIEF STUDY COURSE IN HOMEOPATHY, 3rd edition, Dr Elizabeth Wright-Hubbard, Formur, Inc., St Louis, USA, 1983

CHILDREN'S TYPES, Dr Douglas M. Borland, British Homoeopathic Association, London, UK

CLASSICAL HOMOEOPATHY, Dr Marjory Blackie, eds. Dr Charles Elliot and Dr Frank Johnson, Beaconsfield Publishers, Beaconsfield, UK, 1986

DESKTOP GUIDE TO KEYNOTES AND CONFIRMATORY SYMPTOMS, Dr Roger Morrison, Samuel Clinic Publishing, California, USA 1993

DIGESTIVE DRUGS, Dr Douglas M. Borland, British Homoeopathic Association, London, UK

THE ESSENTIALS OF HOMEOPATHIC MATERIA MEDICA, Dr Jacques Jouanny, Laboratoire Boiron, France, 1980

THE ESSENTIALS OF HOMEOPATHIC THERAPEUTICS, Dr Jacques Jouanny, Laboratoire Boiron, France, 1980

EVERYDAY HOMEOPATHY, Dr David Gemmell, Beaconsfield Publishers, Beaconsfield, UK, 1987

THE HANDBOOK OF HOMEOPATHY, Gerhard Koehler, Thorsons Publishing Group, UK and USA, 1986

HOMOEOPATHIC MEDICINE, Dr Trevor Smith, Thorsons Publishers Ltd, Wellingborough, UK, 1982

HOMOEOPATHY IN PRACTICE, ed. Dr Kathleen Priestman, Beaconsfield Publishers, Beaconsfield, UK, 1982

HOMOEOPATHY: MEDICINE FOR THE 21ST CENTURY, Dana Ullman, North Atlantic Books, Berkeley, California, USA, 1968

INTRODUCTION TO HOMOEOPATHIC MEDICINE, 2nd edition, Hamish W. Boyd, Beaconsfield Publishers, Beaconsfield, UK, 1990

MATERIA MEDICA OF NEW HOMOEOPATHIC REMEDIES, Dr O.A. Julian, trans. Virginia Mundy, Beaconsfield Publishers, Beaconsfield, UK, 1979

THE ORGANON OF MEDICINE, Dr Samuel Hahnemann, 5th edition, trans. R.E. Dudgeon, with additions by William Boericke, Roy Publishing House, Calcutta, India, 1970

THE ORGANON OF MEDICINE, Dr Samuel Hahnemann, 6th edition, trans. J. Kunzli, A. Naude and P. Pendleton, Tarcher Publications, Los Angeles, USA, 1982

THE PATIENT, NOT THE CURE, Dr Marjory Blackie, Macdonald & Jane's, London, UK, 1976

POCKET MANUAL OF HOMOEOPATHIC MATERIA MEDICA, 9th edition, Dr W. Boericke, Boericke & Tafel, Philadelphia, USA 1927

SAMUEL HAHNEMANN, Trevor M. Cook, Thorsons Publishers Ltd, Wellingborough, UK, 1982

Useful Addresses

US HOMEOPATHIC ORGANIZATIONS

Those with 800 numbers may be dialled free of charge within the United States.

HOMEOPATHIC EDUCATIONAL SERVICES
2124 Kittredge Street, Berkeley, CA 94704
510 649 0294; orders 800 359 9051
Provides a general information service and sells homeopathic books, tapes, software, medical kits and medicnes.

HOMEOPATHIC PHARMACOPEIA CONVENTION
Contact Jack Borneman
P.O. Box 80185, Valley Forge, PA 19184
610 783 5124
Supplies a list of manufacturers of homeopathic medicines.

INTERNATIONAL FOUNDATION FOR HOMEOPATHY
P.O. Box 7 Edmunds, Washington, WA 98020
425 776 4147
Promotes the teaching of classical homeopathy to health professionals.

NATIONAL CENTER FOR HOMEOPATHY
801 N. Fairfax #306, Alexandria, VA 22314
703 548 7790
This is the major organization for homeopathy in the USA. The Center is a non-profit membership organization that offers a monthly newsletter, educational programs for the public, training courses for professionals, an annual conference open to the public plus research services for members.

US HOMEOPATHIC PHARMACIES/MANUFACTURERS

Those with 800 numbers may be dialled free of charge within the United States.

BIOLOGICAL HOMEOPATHIC INDUSTRIES
11600 Cochiti S.E., Albuquerue, NM 87123
800 621 7644

BOERICKE & TAFEL
2381 Circadian Way, Santa Rosa, CA 95407
707 571 8202; orders 800 876 9505

BOIRON-BORNEMAN INC.
6 Campus Boulevard, Newton Square, PA 19073
610 325 7464; orders 800 258 8823

BOIRON-BORNEMAN INC.
98c W. Cochran, Simi Valley, CA 93065
805 582 9091

DOLISOS AMERICA INC.
3014 Rigel Avenue. Las Vegas, NV 89102
702 871 7153; orders 800 365 4767

LONGEVITY PURE MEDICINE
9595 Wilshire Boulevard, Beverley Hills, CA 90212
310 273 7423; orders 800 327 5519

LUYTIES PHARMACAL
4200 Laclede Avenue, St Louis, MO 63108
314 533 9600; orders 800 325 8080

STANDARD HOMEOPATHIC COMPANY
154-210 W. 131st Street, Los Angeles, CA 90061
213 321 4284; orders 800 624 9659

Acknowledgements

A–Z Botanical Collection Ltd 89, 116, 156 right; Taeke Henstra/Petit Format 34; Sam Ke Tran 42, 62; BSIP, Alexandra 50; Julia Hancock 58, 122; Rosemary Greenwood 63 top left; Sheila Orme 63 top right, 158; Dan Sams 94, 160; Malcolm Warrington 100, 149; The Picture Store 139; Andrew Brown 141, 171; David C Clegg 147.

Vanessa Fletcher 1, 10, 11, 134
Image Bank, David de Lossy 110
Oxford Scientific Films, Scott Camazine 54, 132, 154; Stan Osolinski 56, 168, G.A. MacLean 107, 138, 153
Zefa 111

Index